INFERTILITY, IVF AND MISCARRIAGE

THE SIMPLE TRUTH

A Guide For The General Public

DR SEAN WATERMEYER
BSC (HONS). MBBCH. MRCGP. FRCOG. MD.
CONSULTANT IN OBSTETRICS AND
GYNAECOLOGY

Edited by Dr Amanda O'Leary
Subspecialist in Reproductive Medicine
CRGW (Centre for Reproduction and Gynaecology Wales)

PARTHIAN

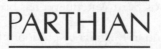

Printed and bound in Bulgaria by pulsioprint.co.uk

ISBN 978-1-912109-64-7

This book is dedicated to all the amazingly courageous patients I have been privileged to serve.

Preface

In the world of infertility, individuals and couples trying to conceive will often have a vast array of questions to ask and they don't always know where or to whom to turn to for help. There is a lot of information available from various sources, particularly the internet, to allow these questions to be answered, but also lots of incorrect information that is fragmented. This sometimes makes it difficult for people to make an informed choice or indeed make the right decisions as they strive to have children of their own.

This book offers the necessary advice and guidance to help you answer these questions. Each chapter is structured around the commonly asked questions and presents the options available in an easy to read and down to earth style.

This book will arm you with everything you need to know and understand about fertility and getting pregnant.

Dr Amanda O'Leary
Subspecialist in Reproductive Medicine
Centre for Reproduction and Gynaecology Wales (CRGW)

***

With people waiting longer to get married and waiting longer to have children, many more people are experiencing fertility issues. In an amazingly clear and concise way this book, which is both easy to read and beautifully presented, gives precise facts clearly and succinctly. This allows patients to easily navigate the often confusing information overload associated with infertility with additional tips to avoid being unnecessarily delayed in their quest of parenthood.

Dr Lyndon Miles
Consultant Embryologist

CONTENTS

ACKNOWLEDGMENTS

I wish to thank my wife, Alison, who has been a wonderful source of encouragement and support. Not only that, she has proofread the book to ensure that it is written in plain English and not complicated medical jargon!

I want to thank my NHS colleagues.

I want to thank all my colleagues at CRGW (Centre for Reproduction and Gynaecology Wales), who have taught me a huge amount. A special mention of Dr. Amanda O'Leary, Mr. Hatel Tejura, Dr. Lyndon Miles, Dr Helen Priddle and Dr Grace Jose.

Foreword

There is within the massive majority of us human beings a deep-seated need to replicate ourselves, to pass on a little of who we are on into the next generation and beyond. It is my opinion that there is a compulsion within our nature to have children to hold, to love, and to nurture. It is as basic as the human need to love and to be loved. In a world where certainties over God, religion and afterlife are becoming ever more abstract, the certainty of living on through one's children is ever more attractive and important.

I remember being surprised at the strength of feeling and turmoil of emotions that I experienced when my partner and I first started to try and have a family. I remember a glimpse of the dread that I felt when the possibility of being unable to have children dawned on me, and then the overwhelming joy at finding out my wife was pregnant and the subsequent elation on becoming a parent.

In my professional life I have unfortunately found that there is much ignorance and misinformation banded about regarding infertility and often couples desperate to have a child are left high and dry. Advice from the internet, friends, or indeed even some medical professionals is at times confusing and on occasions erroneous. In this book designed for the layman, I hope to provide a clearer picture and an answer to many of the questions I am frequently asked in my role as an infertility doctor and consultant obstetrician/gynaecologist.

I am lucky enough to have three wonderful children – what a rollercoaster. Boundless love, joy, tears, anger, pleasure – every conceivable (if you'll forgive the pun) emotion and completely knackering, not to mention hugely costly! I would not have missed a single moment. As a parent and a doctor I wish the very same for each of you and my hope is that this book helps you to achieve it.

Sean Watermeyer

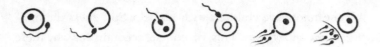

CHAPTER 1

The problem and when to start seeking advice

Introduction

The aim of this short book is to empower you... would-be parents with a basic understanding of the whole process of why couples cannot conceive, what must be done to investigate this, and then what is a sensible plan of action depending on the findings of investigations. More importantly I will endeavour to give you a realistic approximation of your chances of success. Please understand this is not a clinical textbook written for doctors and nurses. It is a manual written by a parent and infertility doctor for the ordinary man and woman. It is written for heterosexuals, for homosexuals, and for loving couples of whatever persuasion who want a child of their own to love and bring up. I only hope I can do it justice and give you, the reader, the information, understanding, and courage to take things forward to achieve your dream.

How big a problem is infertility in the West?

Approximately 1 in 6 couples in the Western World (about

15%) cannot have children without help. So I guess the message is *you are not alone*. This, of course, accounts for why there are so many IVF units in the UK and around the world. The infertility industry is a massive one – this is why you need to make sure you have a basic understanding of the whole process. I see many couples in both the NHS and in private infertility clinics who feel that they have been misled about their inability to have children. Years go by without any active investigation or action and then on occasions it is **simply too late**. Nothing gives me more pleasure, as a clinician, to see understanding on the faces of my patients as they leave the consulting room with a basic understanding and plan of action to help them achieve their dream of becoming parents.

What is the definition of infertility?
Couples often ask the definition of infertility and the simplest answer is… if you have been trying for 1 year or more with no success you may have a problem. Some authorities state 18 months. Obviously to achieve a pregnancy you have to have sex. You may laugh but I do occasionally see couples who sit in clinic and explain that after 1 year they have not managed to get pregnant – but he lives in London and she lives in Scotland, they meet on occasional weekends and hope for the best! Therefore the definition includes 12 to 18 months of *regular* intercourse without using any form of contraception.

How long does it take on average to get pregnant?
Do not be disheartened if the urine pregnancy test kit from the chemist is not positive after a couple of months of trying. On average it is estimated that if it is going to work, approximately 85% of couples have conceived after 1 year of trying. So nature

is not terribly brilliant at getting people pregnant – every month of trying only 5-20% of the time (depending on age) will you become pregnant. That means 80-95% of the time, despite your best efforts, at the end of that cycle the pregnancy test remains negative. So do not be disappointed if you do not get pregnant immediately, particularly if you are young.

How important is age with regard to fertility?
This is a big deal for women. Having said that, time is of the essence. How can I say this nicely? Once women get to the lofty age of 35 years old, their fertility significantly reduces. This also occurs to a much lesser degree with men after the age of 40 years old. Probably one of the most important factors in fertility is the age of the eggs, and this has a major influence on not only whether women get pregnant in the first place but whether they stay pregnant (in other words, the older the woman is, the older her eggs are, the greater the risk of miscarriage).

Age (years)	Natural pregnancy rate per cycle of trying	Miscarriage rate
20s	20-25%	10%
Early 30s	15%	20%
>35	10%	25%
40s	5%	>30%

The above table indicates the chances of pregnancy and miscarriage that are age related. A woman is born with a finite number of eggs and this number reduces over time until there are essentially none left (which is when she goes into menopause) – time for hot flushes (or as the Americans say, "flashes"; somewhat unfortunate when translated into the UK equivalent). Blokes on the other hand continue to make sperm for the majority of their lives. They are not born with a set number of sperm, but produce a new batch approximately every 3 months.

How do I know how many eggs I have left in my ovaries?
The answer is to have a test called an AMH or Anti-Mullerian Hormone. This is a simple blood test that a woman can have at any time of the month (it does not need to be taken at a particular time in a woman's cycle) that gives information on her ovarian reserve. In other words, if there are plenty of eggs in that woman's ovaries the AMH is normal or high; if the number of eggs is starting to dwindle the AMH is low. Your GP will probably not know about this and generally it is not available on the NHS, but you can have it privately (about £80). This is a good test to have for a number of reasons:

  i. If you are relatively young (less than 35 years old) and the AMH is normal it is reassuring that the couple have some time to play with.

  ii. If, however, the AMH is low, then even if that woman is relatively young, the test indicates that her ovarian reserve is starting to deplete and that the sooner action is taken to help her conceive the better. Remember that approximately 1% of women will have completed their menopause by 40 years of age and I have seen and treated a number of women who were menopausal in their late 20s and early 30s – a disaster if they want their own children.

  iii. Finally, if a couple are going for IVF then there is

correlation between the AMH blood test and the number of eggs/embryos that are obtained with IVF treatment.

What should you do if you have a family history of early menopause (Premature Ovarian Failure)?

About 1% of women will start experiencing hot flushes, poor sleep, irregular periods and then cessation of periods before their fortieth birthday. They have likely gone into early menopause or premature ovarian failure (POF). Then, it may be too late to have a baby using your own eggs, even with IVF. In most cases, the reason for POF is called "Idiopathic" – in other words nobody knows why it has happened. In other cases, there are obvious reasons for example a past history of chemo/radiotherapy for a cancer in early childhood. If a medical cause for early menopause is not obvious, then the reason may be genetic.

It is thought that in about 10-20% of women with POF there is already a family history of it in their mother or sister.

If there is a family history of inherited intellectual disability, autism, Ataxia (abnormal balance/co-ordination/speech), learning disabilities, and ADHD (Attention Deficit Hyperactivity Disorder)-like symptoms – then the women may be a carrier of a genetic condition that includes Fragile X Syndrome (FXS), the most common cause of inherited intellectual disability. One important genetic condition associated with early menopause is Fragile X associated Primary Ovarian Insufficiency or FXPOI for short. Some authorities indicate that 1 in 150 women may be "carriers" of the genetic abnormality without knowing it and so be unaware of the possibility of passing it on to their children. **So, if there is a strong family history of the above,**

seek advice and get tested.

I guess then knowing the age at which your own mother went through the menopause is likely to give a clue for the timing of your own menopause. There is evidence that having an AMH blood test may well be a good marker of early ovarian decline even in genetic causes such as FXPOI. **If in doubt – have an AMH blood test.**

Why is the age of the woman and her eggs important?

Up to 90% of eggs / embryos that are produced by a woman **over** 40 years old may be genetically abnormal – this is not to say that the woman or her partner are genetically abnormal, but that the ageing process has an adverse effect on an older woman's eggs. This means natural pregnancy rates are right down and miscarriage rates are right up. This is scary stuff. There are, of course, still women who manage to conceive and carry a baby who are 40 years old – so it is by no means hopeless, **but I want couples to know how important maternal age is in realistically achieving their dream and so how important it is to get help early particularly if the woman is older.**

In a woman over 45 years old, the chance of spontaneous natural pregnancy is less than 1%. If the couple do manage to get pregnant, the risk of miscarriage is over 50%. The reason is that virtually all their eggs are genetically abnormal. I occasionally see women who are coming up to 43-44 years old and I hate it, because I have to tell them that the chance of them getting pregnant with their own eggs is very small… not impossible… but pretty remote. But you can only fix something or sort it out if you deal with the truth. Patients often quote famous women having babies well into their 40s and are disheartened to hear my suspicions that many of them have had IVF using donor eggs (eggs donated from much younger women).

So the message is:

1. Infertility is very common – 1 in 6 couples – you are not alone.
2. If you are young with a normal AMH, to get pregnant naturally can take time – do not despair.
3. Do NOT wait until you are over 35 years old to have children – your fertility significantly reduces and your miscarriage rates go up.
4. Certainly if you have been trying for a year or more to conceive *(regular unprotected intercourse)* and nothing has happened – get medical help. The older you are, the more important this becomes. **DO NOT BE FOBBED OFF.**
5. If there is a family history of early menopause or Fragile X Syndrome, seek medical advice and get tested.
6. If in doubt – get an AMH to ensure that you have good ovarian reserve with the good reserve of eggs.

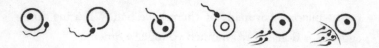

CHAPTER 2

The female body and how it works

Introduction

During the course of this chapter, I just want to go through what I normally say/explain to couples in clinic with regard to what happens during a normal menstrual cycle, the timing and frequency of sex that is required and the natural success rates per cycle of trying. Understanding is the key to identifying the possible simple pitfalls as to why you are not managing to get pregnant.

What do I need to get pregnant?

A normal womb (or uterus) with a healthy endometrium (lining of the womb);

Open healthy fallopian tubes;

One or more ovaries that produce eggs;

Normal mobile sperm;

Regular unprotected sex

A natural cycle – 5 simple steps

Step 1

Following a period, a hormone called FSH or Follicle Stimu-lating Hormone is produced by the female brain. FSH does what is says on the tin – it stimulates the formation of follicles (a follicle is like a small bag-like structure in the ovary that contains an egg). During a natural cycle, FSH stimulates one follicle to grow until it reaches about 18-20mm in size, at which point it is ready to release an egg (ovulation).

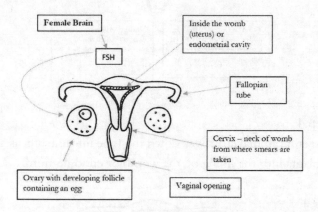

Step 2

The brain releases another hormone called LH (Luteinising Hormone) which stimulates ovulation or release of the egg from the ovary and the egg is picked up by the fallopian tube.

Step 3

The couple have sex and the sperm have to swim from the top of the vagina, through the uterus and into the tube where they meet and one of them penetrates the egg (fertilisation) to form an embryo.

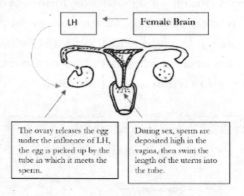

The ovary releases the egg under the influence of LH, the egg is picked up by the tube in which it meets the sperm.

During sex, sperm are deposited high in the vagina, then swim the length of the uterus into the tube.

Step 4

The embryo makes its way down the tube into the uterus and implants into the lining of the womb or endometrium.

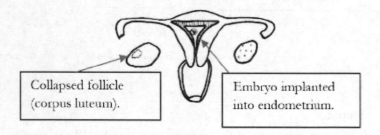

Collapsed follicle (corpus luteum).

Embryo implanted into endometrium.

Step 5

The embryo now starts to grow and releases a hormone called Hcg (Human chorionic gonadotrophin). This is the hormone that causes a pregnancy test to turn positive. The ovarian follicle, having released its egg, collapses on itself and becomes known as the corpus luteum – it is this that produces progesterone. Progesterone stabilises the endometrium (lining of the womb) preventing menstruation so that the pregnancy continues.

If all this works what are the chances of pregnancy for every month of trying?

The chance of a woman becoming pregnant per cycle of trying is between 5-25% depending on the age of the woman. This is not the most efficient of nature's pathways, particularly when having achieved a pregnancy, the miscarriage rate is then 10-30%, again age dependent. Thus if you are a relatively young woman (<35 years old) do not despair if you haven't conceived after 6 months, time is on your side and FURTHER ATTEMPTS should be made. If however you are older than 35 years, I would suggest at the very least having an AMH to ensure good ovarian reserve. If the AMH is low, seek help.

What are the important reproductive hormones that you produce and what do they do?

There are 5 important hormones as follows:

i. FSH (Follicle Stimulating Hormone) – produced by the brain to stimulate the ovaries to produce follicles that contain eggs.

ii. Oestrogen – produced by the ovaries and causes the endometrium to thicken up ready for implantation of the embryo.

iii. LH (Luteinizing Hormone) – produced by the brain to stimulate release of an egg from the ovarian follicle.

iv. Progesterone – produced by the collapsed ovarian

follicle (corpus luteum) after release of the egg to stabilise the endometrium and stop menstruation.

v.   Hcg (Human Chorionic Gonadotrophin) – produced by the implanted embryo and responsible for the positive pregnancy tests. **The purpose of the Hcg is to stabilise the corpus luteum which therefore continues to produce progesterone. Since progesterone stabilises the endometrium you do not have a period and the pregnancy continues.**

When trying to get pregnant can you monitor these hormones to improve timing?

Ovulation kits are available from the chemist – these merely measure LH levels. A raised LH level would indicate ovulation and the couple know then to have sex.

GPs often carry out a "Day 21 Progesterone Test" to see if you have ovulated that month. If you ovulate, the collapsed ovarian follicle or corpus luteum produces progesterone. Therefore if your GP does a blood test in the second half of your cycle and the progesterone level is raised – it is likely that you ovulated that month.

The reason that it is called a "Day 21". Progesterone Test is because in the case of a woman with a 28 day cycle, progesterone levels are found to be highest on day 21. A woman will almost always ovulate 14 days before her period and the progesterone levels will be highest 7 days after ovulation – so in a woman with a 28 day cycle, she will ovulate on day 14 and progesterone will be highest on day 21.

Pregnancy tests are available from the chemist and they measure Hcg levels that indicate if you are pregnant.

If all is normal how can we best achieve a pregnancy?
It is important to remember that **sperm can last up to 6 days in the female genital tract**, and that a released egg can last up to 48 hours. So you do not have to have sex every hour on the hour around the time you ovulate! In fact this can be detrimental to your chances of conception. Remember that the sperm count is at its most potent if ejaculation occurs every 2-3 days. Also remember that ovulation occurs consistently 14 days prior to the start of your period, as long as you have a reasonably regular period.

　Therefore try:

　28 day cycle -

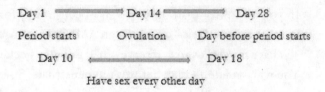

Day 1　　　　　　　Day 14　　　　　　Day 28
Period starts　　　　Ovulation　　　Day before period starts
　Day 10　　　　　　　　　　　　　Day 18
　　　　　　Have sex every other day

　32 day cycle -

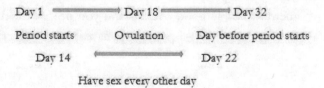

Day 1　　　　　　　Day 18　　　　　　Day 32
Period starts　　　　Ovulation　　　Day before period starts
　Day 14　　　　　　　　　　　　　Day 22
　　　　　　Have sex every other day

Are there any physical signs that indicate ovulation?
Change in Cervical Mucus – your cervical mucus changes around the time of ovulation. It goes from being relatively

thick and scanty to a clearer, more watery consistency, and there is usually more of it.

Basal Body Temperature (BBT) – after ovulation your body temperature rises by about 0.4 degrees. Some women will take their own temperature around the same time every day until a sudden rise, usually midcycle, indicates ovulation.

So the message is:

1. In fertility, there are 5 simple steps to how your body works and 5 main hormones of which to be aware.
2. The chance of getting pregnant naturally per month of trying is 5-25% depending on the age of the woman – so do not despair if you are not pregnant after 6 months of unprotected sex.
3. If you are older than 35 years and been trying for 6 months with no luck – check out an AMH test to ensure you have normal ovarian reserve – If it is low… get help.
4. You will ovulate 14 days before you menstruate. So in a woman with a 28 day cycle you will ovulate on day 14, in a woman with a 32 day cycle you will ovulate on day 18 and so on – this is important for timing sex.
5. Sperm last up to 6 days in the female body after sex, so there is usually good overlap and you do not need to have sex every day – it is better to have it every other day.

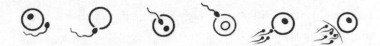

CHAPTER 3

So you can't get pregnant. Why not?

Before I go into what investigations need to be carried out in a couple presenting with infertility, let me firstly go through "What causes Infertility?"

First of all – no blame culture

When I see couples coming through the door of the infertility clinic and settle down into the chairs of the consulting room, there is sometimes what I can only describe as an "atmosphere". One of the couple looks slightly uncomfortable or even sheepish because "blame" for the couple's inability to have a child has already been decided. The very first thing that needs to be done in such circumstances is to remove such "blame" from the equation. Not only is it unhelpful, but can be destructive within the relationship. The path of conception, pregnancy and birth is not an easy one and the couple need to be mutually loving and supportive of each other to succeed in their quest to have a child. Reference to the problem being "someone's fault" will never help and I would therefore ask you to avoid such judgement, using all your energy positively to achieve your mutual dream.

The rule of thirds

There is usually a rule of thirds with regard to why a couple cannot conceive:

1/3 of the time – problem with the woman.

1/3 of the time – problem with the man.

1/3 of the time – unexplained.

In order to get pregnant a woman must have a uterus with a normal lining of the womb (or endometrium), unblocked fallopian tubes, at least one working ovary producing an egg on a regular basis, and unprotected sex at the right time of the month. There is no reason why a woman cannot have a baby with just one ovary, or indeed one open fallopian tube, however, on occasions this may reduce the chances of pregnancy. One third of the time, infertile couples can go through all the investigations outlined below and they are ALL normal. The diagnosis is then one of "unexplained infertility" – these couples generally need help with fertility treatments.

Reasons for Infertility

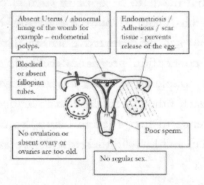

Absent Uterus / abnormal lining of the womb for example – endometrial polyps.

Endometriosis / Adhesions / scar tissue - prevents release of the egg.

Blocked or absent fallopian tubes.

No ovulation or absent ovary or ovaries are too old.

Poor sperm.

No regular sex.

No Uterus/Womb

Evidently if a woman does not have a uterus, she cannot carry a baby. There are a number of reasons for an absent uterus, including having had a previous hysterectomy for all sorts of medical reasons or the fact that the woman was born without a uterus (congenital). This does not necessarily stop a couple having their own child. In fact in the past I have been privileged enough to help a couple in whom the woman did not have a uterus, have their baby. If you still have your own ovaries, it is entirely possible to remove eggs from you using IVF techniques, fertilise your eggs with your partner's sperm and place the resultant embryo into a surrogate (a friend, sister, or altruistic person). They then have your baby for you.

Abnormal Lining of the Womb/Polyps

The lining of the womb or endometrium can on occasions be distorted by small or medium sized outgrowths called polyps that project into the endometrial cavity. It *may* be that these polyps or outgrowths prevent implantation of the embryo or indeed they may even have a role in miscarriage. Removal of these polyps will help with normal implantation and probably reduce the risk of miscarriage.

On occasions there is scarring of the endometrial lining, that can be caused by excessive "curettage" or "scraping" of the endometrial lining during previous operations such as surgical evacuation following miscarriage or termination of pregnancy. Assessment of the endometrial lining by using a fibre-optic camera or hysteroscope that looks into the endometrial cavity is required and sometimes the damaged endometrial lining can be repaired either surgically or by using high dose oestrogen.

Blocked or Damaged Fallopian Tubes

This is quite a common phenomenon and one of the commonest reasons for blocked tubes is **PID (Pelvic Inflammatory Disease).** Most of the time this is caused by genital tract infections such as chlamydia. A large percentage of men and women who have had or indeed have chlamydia are asymptomatic (they do not have any symptoms, for example pain or discharge). Hence the infection is not treated and damage continues. Even after treatment with strong antibiotics, scarring may remain and so one or both tubes may be blocked. Obviously if the tubes are blocked the egg and sperm do not meet and fertilisation cannot occur. Sometimes the sperm will get through, but the fertilised egg does not. In these instances, sometimes the fertilised egg or embryo will implant into the tube itself and an **ectopic pregnancy** results. Hence, in terms of education and awareness the importance of barrier protection to protect against sexually transmitted infection and thereafter **infertility** is hugely relevant. The figures in the table below indicate the approximate rates of tubal infertility after infection.

Table 1. Infection and its relation to tubal infertility:

PID – causing tubal infertility	% of women with severe tubal damage
1st Infection	10-30%
2nd Infection	30-60%
3rd Infection	50-90%

Absent Fallopian Tubes

Some patients have congenitally absent fallopian tubes, although my experience of this is that it is usually only one side that is affected. Previous surgery to remove a fallopian tube (for example for a past ***ectopic pregnancy*** – implantation of the pregnancy in the tube) may have resulted in the tube being surgically removed. If you become pregnant again, having had an ectopic pregnancy in the past, your chance of a repeat ectopic in the remaining tube is significantly increased. ***Therefore you must have an early scan in the event of being pregnant again to ensure that the pregnancy is sitting in the uterus, not the tube.***

In addition, if one or both of the fallopian tubes have become diseased or partially blocked because of infection or inflammation, they can become full of fluid and are then called a "***Hydrosalpinx***" (one tube affected) or if both tubes are affected, "***Hydrosalpinges***" (Hydro – meaning water, salpinges – meaning tubes). Invariably, these diseased fallopian tubes do not function well and fertility is impaired. ***There is evidence that surgical removal of these "Hydrosalpinges" is beneficial if the woman is to have IVF. Potential toxins can leak from these dilated, fluid-filled tubes into the womb during an IVF cycle adversely affecting any transferred embryos. Hence removal of the diseased tubes before IVF appears to improve the pregnancy rate.***

Failure to Ovulate

One of the commonest reasons women fail to get pregnant is because they do not ovulate on a regular basis. Probably the commonest reason women do not ovulate is ***PCOS (Polycystic Ovarian Syndrome)***. Polycystic ovaries can be seen on a Transvaginal Ultrasound Scan. Women with PCOS usually do not have periods on a regular basis. A woman who has a regular period every 28 to 30 days is unlikely not to be ovulating. However, to test for ovulation a "Day 21" Progesterone blood test can be performed – see Chapter 4.

If the ovary is absent, either from previous surgery for ovarian cysts or endometriosis, then obviously an egg cannot be produced from that side.

Another reason for not ovulating regularly is ***abnormal thyroid levels*** – this can easily be tested with another blood test known as ***"Thyroid Function Test" (TFTs)*** and treated as required.

A slightly more uncommon reason for women not to ovulate is because of a small growth in the brain called a "Prolactinoma" which secretes a hormone called ***Prolactin*** – a simple blood test can be done to ensure that this is normal.

Finally, the age of the eggs is a big deal. If you are in your 20s, your chance of conception is 20-25% per month of trying. If you are in your 40s, your chance of conception is about 5% per month of trying.

No Regular Sex

It is not unusual to see couples presenting to a fertility clinic with a history of being unable to have a baby, in whom she lives in London and he lives in Cardiff. When they do see each other they have intercourse, but often it is infrequent and poorly timed with the woman's time of ovulation. It is worth remembering that on average the chance of conception per month of trying, in a couple in whom everything is normal, is only about 10-15%. So if the sex that a couple are having is infrequent and not at the right time, it is likely to take a good deal longer to get pregnant.

Male Factors

Abnormal sperm count is common and is responsible for the infertility in about a third of the cases seen. It is treatable with IVF techniques. In addition, there are other problems encountered by the man including impotence or the inability to have an erection. Please see Chapter 10.

Endometriosis/Adhesions

One of the other common reasons that your fallopian tubes can get blocked is "Endometriosis". Endometriosis in its simplest terms is when deposits of the lining of your womb (endometrium) grow outside the womb. If you have endometriosis, every month that you have a period and bleed through the vagina, also means that any endometriosis in your pelvis will also have grown and bled. Blood in the pelvis is an irritant and inflammation occurs adjacent to the tubes and ovaries causing scarring/adhesions. Adhesions can be described as fibrous strands of glue-like substance that can pull and fuse adjacent tissues. This may result in distortion of the fallopian tubes and ovaries with subsequent infertility.

Ovarian Endometriosis – as well as causing problems with the tubes, Endometriosis can destroy ovarian tissue. "Chocolate cysts" can form in the ovaries. Endometriotic deposits on the ovary bleed at the same time as you menstruate and form pockets of blood within the ovaries. Old blood resembles chocolate – hence the descriptive term "chocolate cysts". In this way endometriosis can destroy ovarian tissue and interfere with ovulation, possibly resulting in problems conceiving.

It is thought that endometriosis may be present in approximately 20-65% of women with infertility, but equally lots of women with endometriosis have already had children. It can be present in very mild to very severe forms. Some women who have endometriosis never have any symptoms, have children and never know they have the disease. Others present to their doctors with severe symptoms of pelvic pain, painful periods, and pain when they have sex. The gold standard to investigate endometriosis is a "Laparoscopy". This is a camera through the umbilicus (belly button) when the patient is asleep with a general anaesthetic. Endometriosis can then be viewed and treated surgically by either excision or ablation (essentially burning it off) or it can be treated medically (see Chapter 9B Endometriosis).

Unexplained Infertility

So what happens if everything is normal? The woman's uterus and endometrial lining is normal AND the woman is ovulating regularly AND the fallopian tubes are open AND the semen analysis is normal AND the couple are having regular intercourse at the right time. If no pregnancy has occurred after 12 to 18 months the diagnosis is of *Unexplained Infertility. In other words, the medical profession does not know why you are not getting pregnant!* This will usually mean that you will need IUI (Intrauterine Insemination) or IVF. *Do not despair – many couples with Unexplained Infertility manage to have a child following IUI or IVF treatment.*

So the message is:

1. Always think about using a condom to protect yourself from infection – because even after 1 attack of chlamydia up to 30% of the time your tubes will become diseased and blocked, rendering you infertile.

2. If you think you have PID (Pelvic Inflammatory Disease) go to your nearest Genitourinary Medicine Clinic (GUM clinic) present in most hospitals and get checked. The earlier you treat PID, the better.

3. If you are worried you have endometriosis, the most accurate way of knowing if you really have it is to do a laparoscopy.

4. Do not wait too long to have your children – when you are 20 years old, your chance of pregnancy is 20-25% per month of trying to conceive. When you are 40 years old, your chance of pregnancy is 5% per month of trying to conceive.

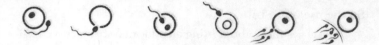

CHAPTER 4

So what investigations do you need?

So now you know the reasons infertility occurs, what investigations are appropriate and can be arranged by your GP or Infertility Specialist?

FOR HER – What basic investigations do I need?

Transvaginal ultrasound scan (TVUS)
One of the best basic investigations for the woman is to have an ultrasound scan of the pelvis. As the name suggests, this is done "transvaginally" by a small probe that goes into the vagina. The uterus, the endometrial lining, and the ovaries can be viewed and abnormalities detected. Fallopian tubes cannot be seen with ultrasound scan because they are too small. If however, the tubes are damaged and full of fluid (known as hydrosalpinx), they become visible on ultrasound.

Are you ovulating? To see whether you are ovulating you can have a "Day 21 Progesterone Test".
This is a simple blood test that measures the hormone progesterone. Progesterone is released after ovulation, so if it is increased you must have ovulated. The timing of the blood

test during your cycle depends on the length of your cycle. The golden rule is that you will almost always ovulate 14 days before you have a period, and if you have ovulated the progesterone level will be highest 7 days after that. So in a 28 day cycle, have your progesterone level measured on day 21 (21 days after the start of your period). In a 32 day cycle, have your progesterone measured on day 25 (25 days after the start of your period).

Are you ovulating? An alternate method to see whether you are ovulating is the "LH Hormone Ovulation test" that can be used at home.

This is a simple kit that you can buy from your local chemist. Essentially when you think you are due to ovulate (instructions are given with the kit), you pee onto a stick. This is then plugged into a small monitor that reads whether you have LH (luteinising hormone) in your urine. You will remember that LH is the signal from the brain for the ovary to release its egg. So if higher levels of LH are detected in the urine it is likely that you are soon to ovulate and sexual intercourse can be timed to maximise your chance of pregnancy. This test may not work so well with women who have polycystic ovaries because they may have elevated levels of LH throughout the cycle.

Are your tubes blocked? To see whether your tubes are blocked you will need a Hysterosalpingogram (HSG).

This is usually done in an X-ray department. You do not need an anaesthetic. During an HSG, a small soft tube or catheter is placed into the neck of the womb or cervix. Dye is pushed into the womb and if the tubes are open, the dye will spill out of the ends of the tubes and into your tummy. An X-ray of the pelvis is taken and will show an outline of the uterus, tubes, and the dye spilling out into your tummy. You then know that your fallopian tubes are open.

Hysterosalpingogram (HSG)

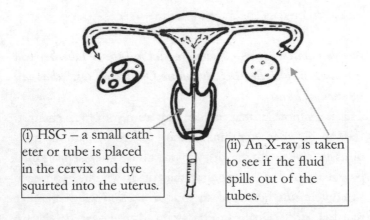

(i) HSG – a small catheter or tube is placed in the cervix and dye squirted into the uterus.

(ii) An X-ray is taken to see if the fluid spills out of the tubes.

Another test to check the fallopian tubes that you may be offered is the "HyCoSy" test or Hysterosalpingo-Contrast-Sonography. Put simply, this is very similar to the HSG test except that it uses ultrasound scanning instead of X-rays. Like an HSG, it is done without the need for any anaesthetic (patients may get some mild to moderate cramping in the pelvis). During a HyCoSy, a small, thin tube is placed into the womb and a substance that shows up on ultrasound scanning is injected. This fills the womb and the fallopian tubes so that tubal patency (open tubes) can be identified when an ultrasound scan is carried out.

Is the lining of your womb normal? To see whether the lining of your womb (endometrium) is normal, you need a hysteroscopy.

A hysteroscopy is essentially introducing a "fibre-optic camera" on the end of a metal rod into the womb to look at the endometrial cavity and occasionally to take a biopsy from it. Sometimes the lining of the womb can be distorted by having small growths called polyps. These can stop the implantation of the embryo into the lining of the womb and so stop you getting pregnant. Alternatively, they may also cause miscarriage. These polyps can be removed either with or after hysteroscopy. A transvaginal ultrasound scan (TVUS) will often show up endometrial polyps or the possibility of "damaged" endometrium. If there is any doubt, direct viewing of the endometrium can be achieved with hysteroscopy.

On occasions I have seen patients who have been unable to have a baby and when the hysteroscopy was done, a polyp (like a skin tag) was sitting within the womb – polyps can prevent the embryo implanting into the endometrium and so stop a woman becoming pregnant. Once the polyps were removed, it is thought that pregnancy can take place.

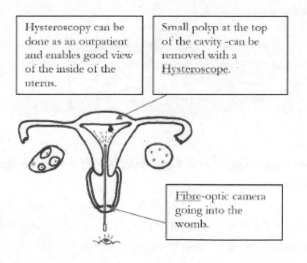

Hysteroscopy can be done as an outpatient and enables good view of the inside of the uterus.

Small polyp at the top of the cavity -can be removed with a Hysteroscope.

Fibre-optic camera going into the womb.

Is your pelvis normal, do you have Endometriosis? To see whether you have Endometriosis or your pelvis is normal you need a Laparoscopy.

During laparoscopy, which is the same as keyhole surgery, a fibre optic camera is placed through the tummy button to directly look into the pelvis. Any Endometriosis or scar tissue can be identified and treated. Also the tubes can be checked to see if they are blocked by squirting blue dye through the cervix in much the same manner as the HSG. If there are no blockages, dye is seen coming out of the ends of the tubes and spilling into your tummy. This procedure needs to be done under a general anaesthetic.

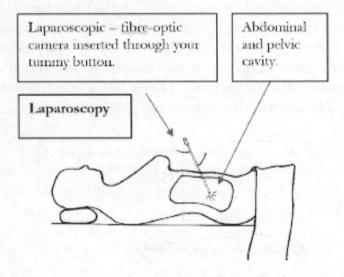

Laparoscopic – fibre-optic camera inserted through your tummy button.

Abdominal and pelvic cavity.

Laparoscopy

How many Eggs have I got left? AMH (Anti-Mullerian Hormone)

AMH is a simple blood test that can be taken at any time of the month within a woman's cycle. It gives information about how many eggs are left in the ovaries of the individual woman having the test. If the AMH is low, then there are fewer eggs left in the ovaries, menopause is closer and timely treatment to aid conception is required. If the AMH is normal or higher, then more eggs are left in the ovaries and menopause is further away. It allows the individual to be slightly more relaxed.

FOR HIM – What Investigations do I need?

THERE IS ONE BASIC INVESTIGATION FOR THE MALE PARTNER

Is your Sperm Sample Normal? Semen Analysis Test

To see whether your sperm is normal you need to have a "Semen Analysis" test. The Semen Analysis test is a microscopic examination of the male ejaculate. Semen is the fluid in which the sperm swim. The specimen should be produced by masturbation into a dry, clean container. This should be examined in the laboratory ideally within 30 minutes of ejaculation. No sex or masturbation should have taken place for three days before the sample is produced. Most fertility units provide a "Semen-analysis Room" (ideally a clean, quiet, comfortable and private room), where the male partner produces his sample. Occasionally the couple will go into the room together where she can provide encouragement to his efforts. If the sample is produced on site the laboratory can examine the sample almost immediately, promoting an accurate result. Sometimes it is difficult for the male partner to provide a sample "on demand" within a fertility unit and he may have to produce a sample at home and bring it in. Within most of these rooms, the Unit provide appropriate pictorial literature to help with the production of a sample.

World Health Organisation (2010) – normal values for Semen Samples:

Volume per ejaculate	1.5ml
Concentration	15 million sperm/ml
Progressive Motility	32%
Normal Forms	4%

What does the above table mean?

a.   The first value is reasonably self-explanatory. You need at least 1.5ml of ejaculate to be normal – some men produce a great deal more than this which is still normal, others less than this which is by the above criteria abnormal and may be the reason for impaired fertility.

b.   The second value refers to the concentration of the sperm within the sample. Again some men have concentrations of sperm up to and beyond 50 million sperm for every ml of ejaculate, but as long as you have at least 15 million sperm for every ml of seminal fluid produced, you are within the normal range. It can be seen that if you produce 1.5ml of ejaculate with a concentration of 15 million per ml, the total number of sperm in the sample will be 22.5 million.

c.   The third value – Progressive Motility – refers to the active *forward* movement of the sperm that can be seen. You may have 100% motility of sperm but if they are all swimming around and around and going nowhere fast, it isn't much good. There has to be progressive forward movement and if a third of your sperm are doing this, you are normal.

d. Finally, Morphology – this refers to what the sperm look like. If they look abnormal or their structure is not right then they have abnormal *Morphology*. Interestingly enough you only need a very small proportion of the sperm to look normal (4% as per the above table), for the sample to be normal.

It is likely that the concentration and progressive motility are the most important values in predicting the chance of pregnancy for either normal sexual intercourse or insemination of the sperm higher into the womb (IUI – intrauterine insemination). Certainly when the concentration is less than 10 million per ml or the progressive motility is less than 20%, normal sexual intercourse or even IUI is unlikely to work and IVF may be a better option. IVF techniques can achieve pregnancy with markedly low sperm counts.

However, it is important to point out that you only need one good sperm in the right place for conception to take place and even if the sperm count is low – although unlikely, it is not impossible for pregnancy to still occur following normal intercourse.

For further reading on Male Infertility, see Chapter 10.

So the message is:

1. Basic investigations include a Transvaginal Ultrasound Scan (TVUS) of the pelvis, D21 progesterone to check if you are ovulating, HSG to check tubal patency, and semen analysis.

2. If you are not ovulating check TFTs (Thyroid Function Tests) and Prolactin, abnormalities of which can prevent ovulation.

3. If there is a suggestion of endometrial polyps on TVUS have a hysteroscopy.

4. If there is a suggestion of Endometriosis consider a laparoscopy.

5. If you have been trying to conceive for 12 to 18 months with no success – do not be fobbed off.

6. Especially if you are nearing 35 years of age, consider an AMH blood test to check your ovarian reserve.

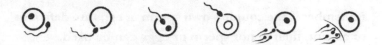

CHAPTER 5A

So what fertility treatments are available and which one do you need?

What fertility treatments are available?

There are essentially 4 main differing treatments that can be used in infertility clinics to help infertile couples get pregnant. Each one is used depending on the underlying reason for infertility. In the event of there being no sperm or eggs available, donor eggs or donor sperm, or sometimes both can be employed.

In addition, if the semen analysis shows that there are no sperm (for example in the case of a man who has had a vasectomy in the past), then a **_surgical_** sperm retrieval can obtain enough sperm for a treatment to achieve pregnancy for that couple.

Clomid with ultrasound monitoring

IUI (Intrauterine Injection)

IVF (In Vitro fertilisation)

ICSI (Intracytoplasmic Sperm Injection)

Use of donor eggs or donor sperm – it is important to

remember if the couple's own sperm or eggs are deficient or absent, then donor sperm or eggs can be used.

Having established the reasons for infertility, what treatment do you need?

Damaged or Absent Tubes – IVF/ICSI

Not Ovulating – *Clomid*/IUI/IVF

Unexplained Infertility – IUI/IVF/ICSI

Poor Sperm Count – ICSI

No Sperm (post-vasectomy) – Surgical sperm retrieval and ICSI or use of donor sperm

Severe Endometriosis – IUI/IVF/ICSI

Same-sex Female Couple – Donor sperm with IUI (D-IUI)/ Donor sperm with IVF (D-IVF)

Absent Womb – IVF/ICSI with a surrogate female

Advanced Reproductive Age/Absent Ovaries – IVF with donor eggs

I will briefly describe each treatment in turn and the reasons behind choosing it.

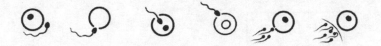

CHAPTER 5B

Clomid with Follicle Tracking

What is *Clomid*?

Clomid is a medication in the form of a tablet. It comes in 50mg, 100mg, or 150mg strengths. Women who are not ovulating for any particular reason or those with established PCOS can use *Clomid* to achieve ovulation and hence pregnancy. *Clomid* works by encouraging the human brain to produce a surge of FSH (Follicle Stimulating Hormone). FSH does what it says on the tin – it stimulates the ovaries to develop follicles which have eggs in them, thereby encouraging ovulation.

How and when do I take *Clomid*?

Day 1 of a woman's cycle is when she starts her period. One tablet of *Clomid* 50mg is taken on a daily basis starting on day 2 and continuing to day 6 (5 days in total during that cycle). This will usually result in a woman ovulating around day 14, hence giving her a 28 day cycle.

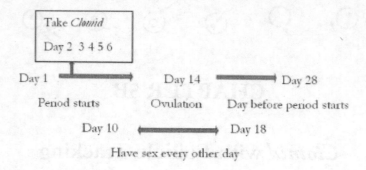

How is the growth of the follicles monitored?

The short answer is with regular ultrasound scans of the pelvis. During a cycle when *Clomid* is used, a series of ultrasound scans are carried out to ensure growth and monitoring of the ovarian follicles. Once a follicle has reached 18-20mm diameter in size, it is likely to ovulate and the couple are advised to have sex every other day to maximise their chance of pregnancy.

How can I better time ovulation?

Once the ovarian follicle(s) have reached 18-20mm (as noted on ultrasound scanning) in size they are mature. At that point, it is possible to induce ovulation with an injection of a hormone akin to LH (it is called *Ovitrelle*). This injection will stimulate ovulation 34-36 hours after it is injected – and so timing of sex can be more precise.

How do I know that I have ovulated?

To ensure ovulation has occurred, a "Day 21" Progesterone level blood test can be taken. If the level is >30mmol/l ovulation is 95% likely to have occurred. Alternatively, follicle tracking with ultrasound scanning can be carried out to image the developing follicle(s) and then the resultant corpus luteum(s) confirming ovulation has taken place.

What happens if I do not ovulate on 50mg of *Clomid*?

If ovulation has not occurred, then the dose of *Clomid* is increased to 100mg during the course of the next cycle. There is probably no advantage in increasing the dose beyond 100mg, although some clinicians will go as high as 150mg.

What are the risks of taking *Clomid*?

The risks of taking *Clomid* include multiple pregnancy (twins ~10-15% / triplets ~1%) and because the ovaries are being pushed to produce follicles then the risk of cystic change in the ovaries goes up. About 10% of women will experience hot flushes.

What happens if I have not had a period so cannot start the *Clomid* on day 2?

If you are not having any periods it is difficult to start *Clomid* on day 2 because you haven't had a period! The answer is to use a progesterone. So if you have not had a period for 2 months or longer, then check a pregnancy test to make sure that you are pregnant. If this is negative, then start a progesterone tablet, such as *Norethisterone* (5mg) three times daily for 5 days. You will remember that progesterone stabilises the lining of the womb (endometrium) so that when it is stopped after 5 days, the endometrium is destabilised and menstruation starts. Count this as day 1, then the following day (day 2) start *Clomid*.

So what are the success rates with *Clomid*?

About 70% of the time, *Clomid* helps non-ovulatory women to produce an egg and if all else is normal with the couple, then up to 50% of couples will have achieved pregnancy within 6 months. Many doctors will use *Clomid* for up to 9 months, if it has not worked by then, other treatments are necessary.

So the message is:

1. If investigations have revealed that you are not ovulating on a regular basis, treatment with *Clomid* is a good and relatively inexpensive first line treatment.

2. *Clomid* does **not** improve your chances of pregnancy if you are already ovulating on a regular basis.

3. If using *Clomid*, insist on having regular ultrasound scans to track the growth of the follicles.

The main risks are those of twin pregnancy and the development of ovarian cysts.

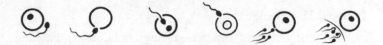

CHAPTER 5C

IUI (Intra Uterine Insemination)

What is IUI?

Intra uterine insemination is exactly that – inseminating the woman with her partner's/donor's sperm into the womb exactly at the time that she is ovulating. This can be done either during a natural cycle or during a medicated cycle when drugs are given to enhance the production of eggs. IUI can be used in patients with PCOS who are not ovulating regularly, in patients with unexplained infertility, in patients with endometriosis who cannot get pregnant naturally. It can be used **_with donor sperm_** in both same sex couples, or indeed in heterosexual couples in whom the partner's sperm is defective or suboptimal.

Reasons for treatment with IUI

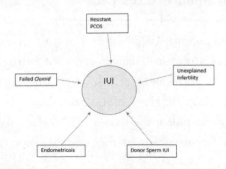

Natural IUI Cycle

Following the start of her period, the woman has a baseline scan to ensure the endometrial lining and ovaries are normal. In a woman with a 28 day cycle, IUI is carried out between day 12 and day 16. A urine or blood test (looking for the rise in LH which indicates ovulation) is used to determine when ovulation has taken place and the partner's/donor's sperm is collected, prepared, and then injected into the womb to coincide with ovulation some 36 hours after the positive ovulation test. A pregnancy test is then carried out about 16 days later.

Natural IUI – need open tubes

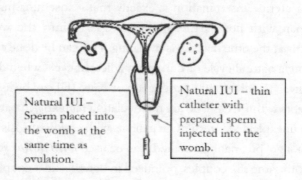

Natural IUI – Sperm placed into the womb at the same time as ovulation.

Natural IUI – thin catheter with prepared sperm injected into the womb.

Medicated/Stimulated IUI Cycle

Following the start of her period, a baseline scan is carried out to ensure the endometrial lining and ovaries are normal. The woman then starts a small daily injection of a drug that closes down her own hormones (see below re: GnRHa/*Suprecur*). A second daily drug (FSH – Follicle Stimulating Hormone) is then given to stimulate the ovaries to produce follicles containing eggs. Regular scans are then carried out to monitor the growth of the developing follicles. When the follicles reach 18-20mm in size they are thought to be ready to ovulate. At that point, a final injection is given (*Ovitrelle*, LH) that causes ovulation. 36 hours later the IUI is carried out.

In contrast to the natural cycle, there may well be more than 1 follicle produced. Most clinics will proceed with the insemination if there are 2 or 3 mature follicles (with 2 or 3 possible eggs) present. However, ovulation of more than 3 follicles with the insemination of millions of sperm is probably not a good idea since the possibility of triplets or quads then goes right up. If too many follicles are produced, it is possible to continue with the insemination if a "Follicle Reduction" is carried out. This is very similar to a transvaginal egg collection carried out with IVF and entails draining unwanted follicles via a needle placed through the vagina under ultrasound guidance to leave 2 or 3 good follicles. The sperm injection or insemination is carried out immediately afterwards.

The insemination itself is a bit like having a smear. It should not be painful. A speculum is inserted into the vagina to see the cervix or neck of the womb. Then a soft flexible tube is inserted into the womb. The prepared sperm is then injected into the womb and hopefully the sperm and egg(s) meet and fertilisation takes place.

What are the success rates with IUI?

Success rates are difficult to judge because women have IUI for all sorts of different reasons. There is some evidence that IUI helps couples to conceive if the diagnosis is (i) Unexplained infertility, (ii) Endometriosis, (iii) Suboptimal sperm counts – although for IUI to have a good chance of success, there must be at least 3-7 million viable sperm injected into the womb.

Success rates with Medicated IUI (partner):

Approx. Take Home Baby Rates – Medicated – **Partner IUI**	
<35 years old	13%
35-37 years old	13%
38-39 years old	10%
40-42 years old	7%
43 years old	Very low%

It is interesting that if ***donor*** sperm (as opposed to partner's sperm) is used, live birth rates with IUI do appear to improve certainly in women less than or equal to 37 years old. So particularly for same-sex couples using donor sperm in an IUI cycle, the table below is more representative:

Success rates with Medicated IUI (donor sperm):

Approx. Take Home Baby Rates – Medicated – **Donor IUI**	
<35 years old	18%
35-37 years old	15%
38-39 years old	11%
40-42 years old	5%
43 years old	Very low%

Before you have IUI, your doctor must ensure that your

fallopian tubes are open and normal otherwise the procedure is a waste of time and money. This can be done with either an HSG test, a HyCoSy or a Laparoscopy (See Chapter 4).

Finally, to qualify for IUI, the male partner must have enough motile sperm in the ejaculate to ensure that after washing and preparation at least 3-5 million motile sperm are delivered into the uterine cavity during the time of insemination. If it is less than this, IVF/ICSI should be considered.

So the message is:
1. IUI is a good initial treatment option for patients with Unexplained Infertility /Endometriosis /PCOS /Failed treatment with *Clomid*.
2. It can be used to achieve pregnancy in same-sex female couples with donor sperm of their choice.
3. The fallopian tubes must have been tested beforehand to ensure that they are open either by HSG or Laparoscopy (keyhole).
4. IUI is cheaper that IVF (about one third of the cost) and so worth considering.
5. If you are not pregnant after 3 treatment cycles of IUI, it is time to move on to possible IVF.

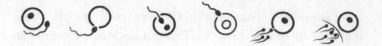

CHAPTER 5D

IVF (In Vitro Fertilisation)

What is IVF?

"In vitro" means "in glass". In other words, fertilisation of the egg and sperm occur outside the body. Fertilisation means the fusing of an egg and sperm to form an embryo. Therefore, IVF is essentially a process where embryos are created outside the body (in a test tube – hence the term "test tube babies").

"In its simplest terms IVF works like this – the woman is started on a daily injection that generally stops her own hormones working. Then an additional daily injection that stimulates her ovaries to produce lots of follicles (containing eggs) is started. After about 10-14 days of growth, these eggs are then removed from the ovaries via a needle through the vagina. The eggs are mixed with the male partner's sperm to form an embryo (test tube baby). The embryo(s) are then placed into a small catheter and placed back in the uterus or womb. Two weeks later a pregnancy test is done".

Reasons for treatment with IVF

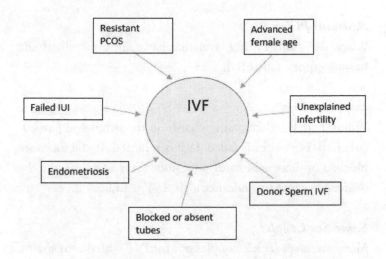

So when is it appropriate to use IVF or ICSI?

Damaged Tubes

Since IVF bypasses the fallopian tubes, any woman with damaged, blocked, or absent fallopian tubes can still get pregnant using IVF. For example – (i) women who have had previous PID (chlamydia) with blocked fallopian tubes, (ii) women who have had previous surgery to remove the tubes because of ectopic pregnancy, hydrosalpinges (dilated damaged tubes) or endometriosis.

Failed IUI

If IUI treatment has failed after 3 cycles, most clinics would recommend the couple to have IVF which has better success rates.

Resistant PCOS
When the woman is not ovulating naturally, especially if she has undergone failed IUI.

Endometriosis
When there is inflammatory change in the pelvis and particularly if IUI has already failed, IVF is required. If the tubes are blocked or there are lots of adhesions (scar tissue around the ovaries) because of endometriosis, IVF is indicated.

Same-Sex Couples
Many same-sex female couples opt for IVF with donor sperm. One of the partners elects to undergo IVF to produce the eggs. These are then mixed with donor sperm to form embryos, which can then be placed back into either of the partners. Often, one of the partners produces the eggs, and the other has the created embryos placed back into her uterus to achieve pregnancy – this way both female partners have a hand in the "making" of their child.

Advanced Maternal Age
Since success rates are a great deal better when using IVF in comparison to IUI, many older women will elect to have IVF. This is because if the age of the eggs is increased OR the AMH is low the chances of pregnancy become lower. So, although it is more expensive to have IVF, it provides the best chance of pregnancy. On occasions, if the woman has a very low AMH, or she is much older, IVF techniques can be used to produce

embryos with DONOR eggs (from a younger woman) – these are then mixed with the partner's sperm to form embryos, one or two of which are placed back into the older woman's womb to achieve pregnancy. This often results in a positive pregnancy test since one of the biggest factors in achieving success, is the **age of the eggs**. If the eggs are from a young woman, the success rates should be good.

Reduced Sperm Counts

If the male partner has a markedly reduced sperm count, then although it is not impossible to conceive naturally or with IUI or IVF, the statistics are not good. Therefore ICSI (see Chapter 5E) is indicated.

Unexplained Infertility

Remember that in 1/3 of couples who cannot get pregnant there is no explanation as to why. These couples will benefit from IVF, especially if the woman is 35 or more years old. IVF can sometimes diagnose why the couple cannot get pregnant – for example about 5% of infertile couples who have never achieved conception together have a problem when the egg and the sperm meet. None of the sperm, despite being present in many thousands, are able to penetrate the egg. In this case IVF can yield eggs, mix them with sperm but nothing happens. These patients need ICSI (see Chapter 5e) when a single sperm is injected directly into the egg to achieve fertilisation.

Step by step guide to IVF (what physically happens)

There are a number of medication protocols or drug treatments used to stimulate the production of eggs but probably the most common treatment is known as the "Long Protocol" and it works like this:

i. After full assessment by medical staff and once the decision for IVF has been made, patients are invited to attend for "treatment planning". This will involve supplying medication (usually in the form of small injections – injected just under the skin, similar to injection of insulin in diabetic patients) and instructions on how and when to give the medication. Generally, the woman or her partner are taught to administer the medication. Dates for the start of your treatment that are mutually convenient are then decided and you are then ready to start.

ii. Twenty-one days after the start of your period, you will be instructed to give yourself a small daily injection (a GnRHa – Gonadotrophin Release Hormone analogue – a common one is "*Suprecur*") that will be continued until the time of your egg collection. A GnRHa is a posh name for a substance that is used to gain control over your natural cycle. It will stop you producing your own Follicle Stimulating Hormone (FSH) and Luteinising Hormone (LH) – this is called "Down Regulation" and means that the fertility clinic can control the growth and collection of eggs at the right time without interference from your own natural hormones. The GnRHa "downregulates" the production of your own fertility hormones.

iii. Usually after 7-10 days of these (GnRHa) daily injections, you will have a period. At that stage you are invited back to the clinic for a "baseline" ultrasound scan. All scans carried out in fertility clinics use the transvaginal route. In other words, instead of the usual scan on your tummy, a slim probe is inserted into the vagina where excellent views of the endometrium, uterus, and ovaries are achieved. At the baseline scan it is important to check that the endometrial lining of the womb is reasonably thin (it should be because you have just had a period and the endometrium has been shed) and that there are no ovarian cysts present. Thereafter, you will be instructed to start the second daily injection (FSH – Follicle Stimulating Hormone) that will stimulate your ovaries to produce follicles (hopefully with eggs in them). Common FSH preparations are called "*Menopur*" or "*Gonal F*". These are small daily injections given just under the skin, but usually in higher doses than you would produce naturally. So instead of just 1 follicle (with an egg in it) being produced as in a natural cycle, multiple follicles in both ovaries are stimulated.

iv. The developing follicles are then monitored with regular ultrasound scans, watching them as they grow. When the maximum number of follicles have grown to around 18-22mm in diameter, they are ready for harvesting. At this point a single injection of LH or Hcg is given in the knowledge that it will result in ovulation 34 to 36 hours later. Therefore a transvaginal egg collection is organised just prior to this in order to collect the eggs before ovulation.

Transvaginal Egg Collection

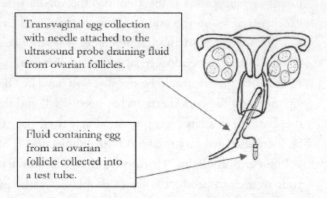

Transvaginal egg collection with needle attached to the ultrasound probe draining fluid from ovarian follicles.

Fluid containing egg from an ovarian follicle collected into a test tube.

The egg collection is usually done under sedation using the equivalent of intravenous *Morphine* and *Valium*, so the patient is sleepy with good pain relief. Some clinics carry out the procedure under general anaesthesia.

v.   Once collected, each egg is then exposed to tens of 1,000s of sperm. Sperm then penetrate the eggs (one sperm per egg) and fertilise them to form the embryos. After their formation, the embryos are generally grown for a further 5 days in the laboratory to reach the "Blastocyst" stage. The embryologist will then choose one or two of the best embryos which are then placed back into the womb. The embryos will need to implant into the endometrium and start to grow. Two weeks later a pregnancy test is carried out.

Embryo transfer

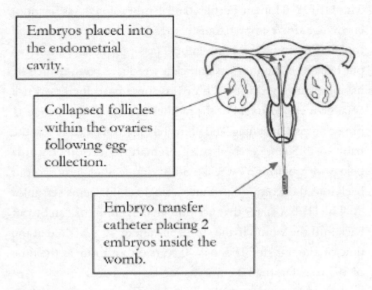

Embryos placed into the endometrial cavity.

Collapsed follicles within the ovaries following egg collection.

Embryo transfer catheter placing 2 embryos inside the womb.

What happens if I have embryos left over?

Frozen Embryo Transfer (FET)

Frequently patients have one or two embryos replaced into the womb, but have embryos left over from their IVF cycle. If these embryos are of good quality they can be frozen and then thawed at a later date for another embryo transfer (known as FET – Frozen Embryo Transfer). The successful thaw rate is approximately 95%. This means that if the fresh embryo transfer failed to yield a successful pregnancy or the couple just want another baby, they can have a FET without having to go through IVF all over again.

How many embryos can be placed into the womb?

The HFEA (Human Fertility and Embryology Association) encourage *single* embryo transfer to reduce the risk of twins and triplets. Put simply, having 1 embryo (as opposed to 2 embryos) put back into the uterus significantly reduces your chance of having twins or triplets. With twins there is an increased risk of almost *everything.* For the mother – miscarriage/diabetes/pre-eclampsia, bleeding, and ultimately maternal death. For the baby – stillbirth, cerebral palsy, prematurity (in other words being born before 37 weeks). So having a single embryo put back into the womb to produce a single child seems sensible.

The HFEA states that no more than 2 embryos can be put back into the womb if the woman is under 40 years old at the time of the transfer. If she is 40 years old or more at the time of the transfer, then 3 embryos can be put back.

It is interesting to note that the **overall pregnancy rates are** **the same** *whether 2 fresh embryos are put back into the womb after egg collection* **or** *1 fresh embryo is put back into the womb after egg collection and if that does not work, a frozen embryo transfer is carried out in a later cycle. The pregnancy rates are the same but the difference is that the significant risks of twins are avoided with the latter.*

How Do I know if my endometrial lining is receptive to the embryo(s) at Embryo Transfer?

A receptive endometrium (lining of the womb) is very important for implantation of the embryo(s) during the course of an IVF / ICSI cycle. As already described it is important to assess the endometrium with ultrasound before IVF to ensure no abnormalities such as polyps or fibroids indenting the endometrial cavity. Sometimes it is necessary to do a hysteroscopy (see Chapter 4). Thereafter, during the IVF cycle, there is some evidence that a thick and juicy endometrium appears to improve pregnancy rates. Some fertility specialists say that *the endometrium ideally should be at least 6mm to 8mm (on ultrasound) in thickness* to ensure a good chance of implantation, although pregnancies can occur even if the endometrial thickness is less than this. In addition, there is some evidence that if the *endometrial lining has a certain "Trilaminar" (3 layered) appearance at the time of the Hcg injection, pregnancy rates are better.* Therefore, during your IVF cycle it is reasonable to ask your fertility doctor about the state of the endometrial lining as they see it on ultrasound.

Finally, if you have had a number (usually 3 or more) of failed implantations, despite having good embryos – there is a relatively new test that looks at the receptivity of the endometrial lining to determine the best time for transfer. *This is called the **ERA** or Endometrial Receptivity Assay.* In addition, there is a procedure called an Endometrial Scratch, carried out in the cycle before your IVF treatment that may improve the pregnancy rates. (Please see chapter 7 for more information on both ERA and the Endometrial Scratch).

Do all the follicles seen on ultrasound scan contain eggs?
Not every follicle will contain an egg. Approximately 70% of follicles drained at egg collection will yield an egg. You cannot see an egg in the follicle on scan. The follicles must be drained and the follicular fluid collected is then viewed under the microscope by an embryologist to identify an egg.

What is a good number of eggs to be collected during an IVF cycle?
The optimal number of eggs to be collected is anything from 4 to 15 during an egg collection. Although what is really important

is not the quantity of eggs retrieved but the quality. I have collected over 10 eggs in some women and they have failed to conceive, whereas others with just 2 or 3 eggs have gone on to have a healthy baby. As a general rule two thirds of eggs collected will fertilise and become embryos. So if 10 eggs were collected, you would expect 7 of them to fertilise to form embryos. Once more than 15 eggs are collected the risk of ovarian hyperstimulation starts to go up (see Chapter 6 – Risks Associated with IVF).

How successful is IVF?

IVF success rates per cycle in the majority of women are approximately 20% to 35%. In comparison, a young fertile couple trying to conceive naturally have a 15% to 20% chance of conception per month of trying. IVF success rates vary depending on the age of the woman and her AMH. Also if she has had a baby in the past, success rates seem to improve.

Be careful to distinguish between "Take Home Baby Rates" and "Pregnancy Rates". Many women will get pregnant with IVF, but this does not equate to a baby in your arms because of the risk of miscarriage. The bottom line is not pregnancy rate, but "Take Home Baby Rate (THBR)". Below is a table giving approximate THBRs depending on age:

Approx. Take Home Baby Rates	
<35 years old	32%
35-37 years old	27%
40-42 years old	21%
43 years old	5%

From this very important table, you can see that a couple will spend approximately £5,000 on a treatment that at best will give them the result they want about a third of the time. If the woman is 43 years old, the couple will spend significant amounts of their income on a procedure that is likely to fail 95% of the time!

It is therefore massively important that the couple are aware of these statistics before investing physically, psychologically, and financially into Assisted Reproduction treatments.

What is IVF Lite?

IVF Lite is a milder form of IVF, using lower doses of drugs for shorter time periods and co-ordinated within the natural menstrual cycle. The focus is on quality of eggs and embryos as opposed to the quantity of eggs and embryos. Some authorities believe that using lower doses of drugs may increase the quality of eggs and embryos, as well as achieving better implantation. In addition, the cost of the treatment is lower because IVF Lite involves less drugs. Risks such as Ovarian Hyper-stimulation Syndrome (OHSS) are lower because the ovaries are not being overly stimulated.

In one particular American study, it was shown that minimal stimulation IVF gave similar results to conventional IVF but was much cheaper with fewer side effects. The same study suggested that in older women and those with very low ovarian reserve, IVF Lite was actually superior to conventional IVF, although for younger women it was slightly worse. The pregnancy rate per egg retrieved in all cases was higher with less stimulation, although of course fewer eggs are likely to be retrieved with IVF Lite.

So the message is:

1. IVF success rates are dependent on many factors including age, AMH, and whether you have had a child before, but in a woman less than 35 years of age, success rates vary between 20-35% per cycle.

2. IVF is the indicated treatment if the tubes are blocked.

3. IVF is the next step if IUI has failed.

4. Consider going straight to IVF if you are older (> 35 years old or your AMH is low).

5. If you have enough eggs – you may have enough embryos for a fresh embryo transfer and still have embryos to freeze – this means you can have a FET (Frozen Embryo Transfer) later on without having to go through a whole cycle of IVF again.

6. For same-sex couples – Donor sperm + IVF is an effective treatment.

7. Ask your fertility clinic doctor about your suitability for IVF Lite.

8. Even if using IVF – success rates drop dramatically with increasing female age – **DO NOT WAIT TOO LONG**.

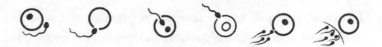

CHAPTER 5E

ICSI (Intra-Cytoplasmic Sperm Injection)

What is ICSI?

ICSI or Intra-Cytoplasmic Sperm Injection is exactly the same as IVF except that following the egg collection instead of each egg being exposed to thousands of sperm, a single sperm is injected directly into each collected egg in the hope that fertilisation will take place and the embryo will form. The inside of the egg is called the *cytoplasm*, hence the term Intra-*Cytoplasmic* Sperm Injection.

Intra-Cytoplasmic Sperm Injection

EGG following transvaginal egg collection.

Cytoplasm inside unfertilised egg.

Single sperm being injected into the cytoplasm of the collected egg.

Hence, if you only have a few sperm (instead of the usual millions of sperm generally required), then ICSI is used. The normal sperm sample will produce 15 million sperm per ml, but with ICSI even if just a few reasonable sperm are produced, the couple can still have a baby.

In addition, if you have had a previous IVF cycle where approximately 40,000 to 100,000 sperm were placed with the eggs but none penetrated the eggs (so there was no fertilisation and no embryos formed) – then a sperm must be directly injected into each egg – in other words ICSI must be utilised.

Following Injection of the sperm, the hope is that fertilisation takes place and embryos are formed. Thereafter, one or two of the embryos are placed into the womb (embryo transfer). Implantation of the embryos into the endometrium then hopefully takes place and a pregnancy test is carried out 2 weeks later.

Reasons for treatment with ICSI vs IVF

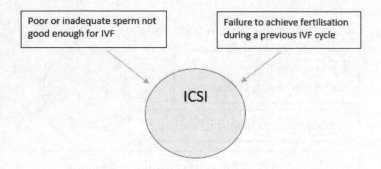

When is it appropriate to use IVF or ICSI?

The reasons to use ICSI as a fertility treatment is exactly the same as for IVF plus 2 factors:

i. Reduced sperm counts – If the male partner has a markedly reduced sperm count then ICSI is indicated. Remember that for IVF you need 1,000s of sperm per egg collected to achieve the formation of an embryo. With ICSI you need 1 sperm injected directly into the egg! So ICSI is used in couples where the man has only a few sperm available.

ii. Failed fertilisation at IVF – About 5% of infertile couples who have never achieved conception together have a problem when the egg and the sperm meet. None of the sperm, despite being present in many millions, are able to penetrate the egg. So when the couple undergo IVF, despite obtaining millions of sperm and a good number of eggs, when they are placed together the sperm are unable to penetrate the eggs and so no embryos are formed. In cases like this the sperm needs to be directly injected into the egg to achieve fertilisation and the formation of an embryo and so ICSI is required. Hence when undergoing fertility treatment, some couples opt to have 50% of the eggs fertilised by IVF and 50% fertilised by ICSI. This means that if there is no fertilisation with IVF, the ICSI backup will still provide embryos.

So the message is:

1. ICSI is the same procedure as IVF, except that instead of thousands of sperm being placed with each collected egg, 1 sperm is directly injected into each egg to achieve fertilisation.

2. There are 2 reasons for using ICSI instead of IVF and they are markedly reduced numbers of sperm and failed fertilisation in a previous IVF cycle.

3. When undergoing an IVF/ICSI cycle, some couples opt to have 50% of the eggs fertilised by IVF and 50% of eggs fertilised by ICSI. This means that if the IVF does not work (no fertilisation), the ICSI backup will still hopefully yield embryos.

4. Success rates are similar to IVF – but again the message is that success rates with ICSI drop dramatically with increasing female age – ***DO NOT WAIT TOO LONG*** before seeking help.

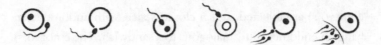

CHAPTER 5F

Advice following your embryo transfer

Couples often ask for advice following their embryo transfer, worried that certain activities may harm the implantation/growth of the embryos or that they may compromise the chances of success – here are a few basic dos and don'ts:

Can I pass urine after my embryo transfer (ET)?

The answer is categorically yes! Many women are afraid to have a pee after ET, because they understandably feel that they may wash the embryos out. Be reassured – this is impossible. The urine is stored in the bladder and exits through a small tube called the urethra. It is completely separate from the cervix and the womb, where the embryos have been placed. Pee to your heart's content, the embryo(s) are safe.

Can the embryo(s) fall out after ET?

When the ET is carried out the embryo(s) are usually placed 1cm to 1.5cm from the top of the womb, inside the womb cavity. But the womb cavity is not a voluminous space into which the embryo(s) are injected. It is a closed space, with endometrium lying on endometrium, analogous to a sandwich. The embryo(s) are then placed in between the layers of the endometrial "sandwich". It is most unlikely that they can fall out.

What should I eat/drink?
It is sensible to eat a healthy, balanced diet. Try to eat plenty of protein and avoid spicy foods and bowel irritants. Drink about 2 litres of fluid per day and avoid caffeine/alcohol. Ensure that you are taking Folic Acid and continue this up to 12 weeks of pregnancy. Continue your medication as per the instructions of your IVF clinic.

Physical activity – what can I do?
Certainly for the first 3-4 days after ET, try and keep physical activity to a minimum, thereafter live life normally but avoid strenuous exercise and swimming certainly until the outcome of the treatment is known. Avoid sex until the outcome of the treatment is known.

Avoid stress
Although, to the best of my knowledge, there is no compelling evidence for this – it is sensible to avoid stressful situations in either in work or at home.

What happens if I have a bleed after the Embryo Transfer?
Light vaginal bleeding can occur following implantation of the embryo, so not all vaginal bleeding is bad news – women can sometimes bleed quite heavily and still be pregnant, so the best advice is to carry on with the above and your medication until the pregnancy test on day 14-16 following the ET. If you

bleed very heavily, however, or have what feels like a normal period – the pregnancy test is likely to be negative.

Once the pregnancy test is positive and then I have a bleed, how do I know if I have miscarried?

Bleeding in early pregnancy is quite common and does not necessarily mean the end of the pregnancy. Once you get to 5-6 weeks gestation, contact your clinic or GP who can organise an ultrasound scan. I have scanned many women who have had bleeding in early pregnancy and the scan findings still showed a normal pregnancy inside the uterus. Even after vaginal bleeding, if a foetal heart is seen on ultrasound – approximately 90% of those pregnancies continue.

However, if a woman experiences pain as well as bleeding in early pregnancy it is likely that she is miscarrying. If this occurs seek MEDICAL HELP, especially to rule out an ectopic pregnancy (pregnancy implanted into the tube) which can be life threatening.

What medication is used after ET?

Commonly, *Progesterones* are used following ET. These medications act by stabilising the lining of the womb and there are a number of different types:

i. Utrogestan 200mcg pessaries – these are usually placed in the vagina, x3 per day until 12 weeks of pregnancy.

ii. Cyclogest 400mcg pessaries – these are usually placed in the vagina x2 per day until 12 weeks of pregnancy.

iii. Gestone Injection (50mg) – this is a daily injection until 12 weeks of pregnancy. It is an Intramuscular injection (deep into the muscle) and it is my experience that women find it more painful to administer than preparations that are subcutaneous (injected just under the skin).

iv. Lubion Injection (25mg) – this is a daily injection until 12 weeks of pregnancy. It is a subcutaneous injection (injected just under the skin) and it is my experience that it is less painful to inject than intramuscular injections.

Some patients **may** also be given other medication which are individually tailored depending on the patients' history and circumstances. They include:

i. *Clexane* (40mg) injections daily if history of miscarriage.
ii. *Prednisolone* (5-10mg tablets daily) if history of miscarriage.
iii. *Oestradiol* (2mg tablets) – if there is a history of poor thickness of the lining of the womb.

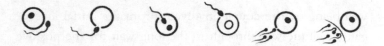

CHAPTER 6

Risks Associated with IVF/ICSI

I wrote this chapter, because from time to time I see couples who merrily waltz into clinic with an unrealistic idea that modern medicine and fertility techniques can sort out any problem and cure any ill – this is just not true. Expectations can be massively high and disappointment completely unexpected. Whilst it is true that millions of IVF babies have been born since the birth of the first IVF baby (Louise Brown) in 1978, it is also true that IVF can be a difficult path to tread where more often disappointment exceeds joy. If you are contemplating infertility treatment do so from a realistic and well informed perspective.

Psychological, Physical and Financial Trauma

Infertility Treatment… "*If successful there are very real and joyful rewards. Even if unsuccessful IVF often draws a line in the sand, after which a couple can reflect, 'we can sleep easy knowing that we tried everything to have our own child'.*" *But there are very real psychological, physical, and financial implications and risks.*

The whole process of going through a fertility treatment has very real implications for the psychological and physical well-being of the couple involved. From the initial investigations all the way through to the long wait for the positive pregnancy test. The journey may involve surgery, for example to remove a polyp from the lining of the womb or indeed an ovarian cyst, and this is before the IVF treatment has even started. The use of medication to stimulate the ovaries is not without its risks in terms of not only general discomfort but also more serious scenarios such as Ovarian Hyper-stimulation Syndrome (OHSS). The transvaginal egg collection carries risks of bleeding and infection, as well the discomfort of a needle into the pelvis and ovaries. The drugs used to either sedate or anaesthetise during the egg collection can induce nausea and vomiting. On occasions the embryo transfer itself can be traumatic, particularly if there is difficulty negotiating the cervix to place the embryo(s) into the correct place within the womb.

The psychological stress on the couple undergoing IVF can be enormous. The drugs themselves can make the woman emotionally vulnerable. Ultimately the necessary exposure of your most personal, intimate self – both psychologically and physically – can be hugely unsettling. The waiting for results of investigations, the understandable fear of various procedures such as egg collection, and then the wait and hope for a positive pregnancy can all be hugely stressful. The cruelty of a positive pregnancy test followed by a miscarriage is a massive kick in the teeth when the couple are already on an emotional rollercoaster. The whole process can put a strain on personal relationships, induce feelings of depression, and inevitably on many occasions tears are shed.

There are important financial implications too. In the UK, the average cost of an IUI treatment is £1,000 per cycle. The cost of an IVF treatment cycle can be anything from £3,500 to £6,000. If ICSI is required, a further £700 to £1,200 can be added to the cost. Following an IVF treatment cycle, if there are embryos suitable for freezing, then a future FET (Frozen Embryo Transfer) will cost approximately £795 to £1,300. So it is important to point out that as well as the physical and psychological trauma, there will be a financial hit as well. My experience of this is that you need to be savvy. Know what your limits are and stick to them. Be careful about possible hidden extra costs, for example like cost of drugs/embryo storage/ extra embryology techniques like assisted hatching. Ensure that hidden costs are exposed so that total expenditure can be assessed and budgeted for. Finally, if you are lucky enough to live in the UK, remember that you are entitled to free NHS fertility treatment (although this is postcode dependent), although that entitlement may change if you have had private treatment. It is also important to know *same sex female couples may well be entitled to NHS Donor sperm-IUI or Donor sperm-IVF*. Often the couples concerned are not aware of this. More worryingly, their GPs are often not aware either.

The Risk of Failure of Treatment

At the risk of sounding like a merchant of doom and gloom, it is important to point out that on average, even in the best hands IVF will yield a "take home baby rate" of about 33%. That means approximately two thirds of the time, an IVF cycle will not work. It is also important to point out that when a clinic publishes its pregnancy rates, this does not equate to the all-important "take home baby rate". This is because of the risk of miscarriage. This, on average, affects between 15-20% of all pregnant women and goes up significantly with age.

Ovarian Hyper-stimulation Syndrome (OHSS)

What is OHSS and how often does it occur?
OHSS is a real problem with infertility treatment and a potential nasty side effect particularly in young women with Polycystic Ovarian Syndrome. It is essentially overstimulated ovaries from the gonadotrophins (FSH) used to stimulate the formation of follicles in the ovaries. The overall approximate risk of getting OHSS is about 4%. The severest form requiring admission to hospital happens in about 0.5% to 1%.

What are the Symptoms of OHSS?
In OHSS, the ovaries become enlarged and the blood vessels in the body become leaky. This results in fluid leaking out of the blood vessels into the abdomen and sometimes lungs. The abdomen can then become swollen and tense, leading to discomfort and sometimes pain. Hence women experience bloating, nausea, and vomiting. Occasionally fluid leaks out into the lungs to cause breathlessness. In addition, women with OHSS are more likely to get blood clots in their legs, arms, neck, or even head, resulting in pain in the affected area or even headache.

How many types of OHSS are there and how long will it last?
There is early or late OHSS. Early OHSS occurs shortly after egg collection (3-7 days). Late OHSS happens following a pregnancy test (12-17 days) and is usually more severe and associated with pregnancy (which causes ongoing stimulation of the ovaries by producing Hcg). The OHSS can last from a few days to a few weeks.

Can OHSS cause death?

The short answer is yes, but it is very rare – approximately 1 in every 425,000 IVF cycles.

How is OHSS treated?

Following IVF/ICSI or even stimulated IUI cycles, if you get any symptoms of bloating, abdominal pain, nausea or vomiting seek help from the clinic where you had your treatment. The HFEA (Human Fertilisation and Embryology Authority) stipulate that patients having IVF should have 24 hours a day access to help. Most cases of OHSS are very mild and resolve with ensuring that adequate fluid is drunk (at least 2 litres of fluid per day) and high protein diet/drinks. Sometimes painkillers/anti-sickness medication is required. Many patients are given a "blood thinner" injection (*Clexane*) which prevents the formation of blood clots. If OHSS is severe, admission to hospital with intravenous fluids, blood tests, and strict monitoring is required. Occasionally, the fluid in the abdomen builds up too much it will need to be drained by thin tube inserted into the abdomen.

If a woman is high risk for OHSS, how can it be avoided?

The risk of OHSS can be reduced by using low doses of gonadotrophins (FSH), particularly in younger women or those with a previous history of OHSS. If during the cycle there are multitudes of follicles with free fluid seen in the abdomen on ultrasound, the cycle can be abandoned. Alternatively the cycle can continue and egg collection can be carried out but all the embryos are frozen. By avoiding a fresh embryo transfer, the patient cannot get late OHSS (usually the more severe form) and then the embryos can be safely frozen and replaced at a later date (as a FET - Frozen Embryo Transfer) when everything has settled down.

Will OHSS affect future cycles?

If you have experienced previous OHSS, then the drug regime used in any subsequent cycle will need to be carefully chosen and the patient monitored even more closely during that cycle. Sometimes the patients are pre-warned that frozen embryo transfer may be more likely in any subsequent IVF cycle.

Risk of Egg Collection

During collection, a needle is inserted through the vagina into the pelvis which forms part of the abdominal cavity. As well as the ovaries and uterus, loops of bowel are present and the operator must take care not to needle the bowel. In addition, there are a number of large blood vessels adjacent to the ovary and any needle must stay well clear of these structures.

Risks are therefore those of potential bleeding and infection. Very rarely, following an egg collection a laparotomy (operation involving surgical opening of the abdomen) is required to fix any potential problems caused by egg collection. Many fertility clinics will give antibiotics prior to egg collection to prevent infection.

There are occasions where the ovaries are so high that they cannot be safely accessed using the transvaginal route. This is why the baseline scan is so important to ensure that the ovaries are accessible.

Multiple Pregnancy

In the UK, the transfer of more than 2 embryos in women under the age of 40 is not allowed. Guidance from relevant

UK authorities encourages single embryo transfer where at all possible. The reason for this is that multiple pregnancies carry significantly increased risks in comparison to singleton pregnancies.

What are the risks in an early twin pregnancy?
Increased risk of late onset OHSS.

Around 30% of twin pregnancies reduce to singleton pregnancy – in other words one of the babies dies.

What are the risks later on in a twin pregnancy?
The perinatal mortality (death rate) and morbidity (disease or disability) rates in twins are approximately 5 times that of singleton pregnancies. Preterm delivery (earlier than 37 weeks) is 3 times more common with twins than with singletons and a major problem with preterm delivery is Respiratory Distress Syndrome (breathing difficulties).

The risk of stillbirth in twins is approximately twice that of singleton pregnancies. There is a fourfold risk of cerebral palsy in twins with increased risks of brain haemorrhage and asphyxia. There is a greater risk of congenital abnormalities in twins.

For the mother the risks go up as well. There are increased risks of anaemia, high blood pressure, pre-eclampsia, abnormal bleeding during the pregnancy, postpartum haemorrhage, and birth complications. Because of the much greater risks to mother and babies, twin pregnancies are always under the care of a consultant obstetrician in the UK and the pregnancies need much greater monitoring with regular scans and antenatal follow-up.

The psychological consequences for families then having

to come to terms with handicapped children and the effect that it has on the immediate and wider family should also be taken into account.

What about triplets and beyond?

Hopefully you have got the picture with regard to the increased risks of twins. With triplets and beyond, the risks go up even more. In fact in some countries, "Foetal Reduction" or the killing of one or more of the foetuses at the end of 12 weeks of pregnancy is carried out to reduce the risks. This can cause miscarriage in up to 15-25% of cases.

How can I reduce my risk of multiple pregnancy?

This is easy – have a single embryo put back. It is also true to say that if the remaining embryo(s) are good enough to freeze and the woman comes back at a later date for a frozen embryo transfer – THE OVERALL PREGNANCY RATES ARE THE SAME.

Risk of congenital abnormality

Are children born by ICSI more likely to have genetic abnormalities/birth defects?

In the UK, thousands of babies are born by IVF, in fact IVF accounts for about 2% of the total number of births and the vast majority of these babies are fine. However, the above question is often asked by couples coming for fertility treatment and the short answer appears to be, yes. ICSI is still a relatively new procedure (started in the UK in the 1990s), but there does seem to be evidence of an increase in abnormalities in children born to parents having either IVF or ICSI. In the UK approximately

2-3% of babies are born with a congenital defect. Major defects include abnormalities of the limbs, heart (for example – a hole in the heart) and spinal cord (for example – spina bifida).

The evidence suggest an approximate doubling of this background risk in terms of a major birth defect with ICSI. However, this still means that if this evidence is correct, 95-96% of the time there will be no major defects. There also appears to be a lesser increase in the risk of minor congenital defects.

When ICSI is used because of abnormal sperm (patients with very low sperm counts), there does appear to be an increase in abnormalities of the sex chromosomes of children born (approximately 1 in 700) and sub-fertile men with specific chromosomal abnormalities may pass on the same fertility problems to their sons. Some men with very low unexplained sperm counts may also be carriers of the cystic fibrosis gene. This means that although they themselves do not have the cystic fibrosis disease, they may pass on the defective gene to any offspring. If their partner also has the defective gene, then any resulting children may inherit the actual cystic fibrosis disease. Hence, it may be sensible for men who have very low, unexplained sperm counts to consider genetic testing.

What can I physically do to reduce the risk of congenital abnormality?

There is evidence that smoking cigarettes, drinking alcohol, and using recreational drugs in pregnancy can increase the risk of congenital abnormalities – SO DON'T.

The first 12 weeks of a pregnancy is probably the most important time to avoid medication and drugs. This is because it is during this time that the internal organs of the developing baby are being formed. After 12 weeks most of the major structures are already formed and now only have to grow. If possible it is always advisable to consider a reduction or stopping some types of medication during the first 12 weeks of pregnancy, *but only after consultation with your doctor.*

Plenty of rest is important. Healthy diet and light exercise is good. Avoid vitamin supplements not designed for pregnancy – for example vitamin A in excessive amounts has been found to cause congenital defects.

Finally, I always ask patients to ensure that they are on Folic Acid. There is evidence that this significantly reduces the risk of conditions like spina bifida in unborn babies. It needs to be taken before conception to make sure that it is in the system, as well as during early pregnancy.

Antenatal Care

Are pregnant women who have had infertility treatment high risk patients?

The answer is categorically yes. In patients who have had IVF, or even just a past medical history of infertility, there is an increase in the risk of smaller, growth-retarded babies, early delivery (prematurity), and stillbirth in comparison to women who have conceived spontaneously.

Should pregnant women conceived by IVF be under Consultant led care?

In view of the above, the answer is yes. Additionally, it is my opinion and practice to ensure growth scans are carried out in such women to ensure that the unborn baby's growth and wellbeing is monitored. The risk of stillbirth goes up with increasing gestation – so that stillbirth is more common at 41 weeks then it is at 39 weeks. Also stillbirth is increased with increasing maternal age. Hence, it is also my practice to ensure delivery of these patients between 39 and 40 weeks – but not later.

So the message is:

1. Infertility treatment is not without its risks. It is costly, physically and psychologically draining.

2. Be realistic – approximately two thirds of the time, each IVF cycle will not work and the success rate declines with age.

3. Since twin or triplet pregnancies are much higher risk than singleton pregnancies, carefully consider having a SINGLE embryo transfer to reduce this risk.

4. Be aware that there is an increased risk of congenital abnormalities in babies born by IVF/ICSI, but the vast majority of babies born are still normal.

5. Do not be fobbed off with suboptimal antenatal care – IVF pregnancies are high risk and regular growth scans throughout pregnancy and delivery at or before 40 weeks should be considered.

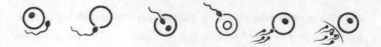

CHAPTER 7

What else can I do to improve my chance of a successful IVF outcome?

On the internet and in the fertility literature there are all sorts of suggestions to improve your chances of conception, and I wanted to simplify these with a few words on each.

Endometrial scratch

This really is what it says on the tin – a scratch of the lining of the womb. The woman has a speculum placed into the vagina (just like when you have a smear) and a thin straw-like tube (called a *Pipelle*) is inserted through the cervix into the womb. The end of the *Pipelle* has a small sharp opening which essentially "scratches" the endometrium, traumatising it in the process. The procedure is carried out in the second half of the cycle (day 19-26) prior to the forthcoming treatment cycle. It is always sensible to take some painkillers (e.g. *Paracetamol* or *Ibuprofen*) about 1 hour beforehand. The procedure is done in clinic, takes about 5 minutes, and you go home about 20 minutes afterwards. Because the lining of the womb is being scratched sometimes you can experience some bleeding vaginally – this is not uncommon and nothing to worry about. In order to have this procedure you need to make sure that you are definitely not pregnant for obvious reasons.

So why do it? It is thought that one of the factors that prevents pregnancy is failure of the embryo to implant into the lining of the womb – this may be because of a poor quality endometrial lining. If a couple produce good quality embryos and then IVF consistently fails to make the woman pregnant it seems logical to assume that the problem may be with the endometrial lining. There have been several studies in the scientific literature to show that endometrial scratching can improve the implantation rate in women with repeated IVF failures. One recent study showed a *20% improvement* in live birth rates.

So if you have had several failed IVF attempts especially with good quality embryos, then it is worth considering an endometrial scratch.

Endometrial Receptor Assay (ERA)

For patients who have experienced recurrent implantation failure following Embryo Transfer, there is a relatively new personalised test that looks at how receptive the lining of the womb or endometrium is for implantation of the transferred embryo(s). The test involves taking a biopsy (just like an Endometrial Scratch) of the endometrium at different times during a woman's natural cycle or during a medicated cycle and analysing it genetically, to determine if it is "receptive" or "non-receptive" for implantation of an embryo. If the endometrium is "non-receptive" at a particular time, the test can be repeated on a different day in the cycle to see when it is "receptive". Once this is known, a frozen embryo transfer or donor embryo transfer can be planned for this "receptive" day in a subsequent cycle.

This technology may help to optimise the timing of embryo transfer, particularly in women who have had recurrent implantation failures.

Intra-lipids

This is basically a bag of liquid fat that is given intravenously (a drip in the arm) around the time of your IVF treatment and post embryo transfer. The theory is that this treatment reduces the NK (Natural Killer) cell population which some people say might affect implantation and miscarriage. There have been clinical studies that have shown improved pregnancy and live birth rates in women having IVF who have had recurrent implantation failure/miscarriage and who have increased NK cells. It is given "off label" (in other words, *not* like a normal prescription) and the Royal College of Obstetricians and Gynaecologists do ***not recommend*** it. It can be associated with severe reactions, thrombosis, and infection.

Have it if you want or alternatively go and have a "fat-boys" breakfast instead.

DHEA (Dehydroepiandrosterone)

DHEA (Dehydroepiandrosterone) exists as a natural hormone in the body that is relatively abundant in the body at around the age of 21 and then significantly drops in concentration with increasing age. DHEA is one of the building blocks or precursors to a number of important hormones needed for reproduction. Since DHEA drops with age and is related to hormone production, researchers have wondered if fertility is improved by taking DHEA supplements particularly in older women.

One study found that by taking three 25mg tablets of micronized DHEA for 3 months before starting IVF stimulation, there was a significant increase in the pregnancy rate. The results suggested an improved ovarian function in poor responders and those over 40 years old by taking DHEA. There is also evidence that DHEA reduces chromosomal abnormalities if taken as a supplement one to three months prior to IVF, which may reduce the risk of miscarriage.

So DHEA taken as the micronized form 75mg daily for 3 months prior to IVF treatment may:

i.   Increase IVF success rate

ii. Increase egg/embryo numbers

iii. Decrease spontaneous miscarriage rates

iv. Reduce chromosomal abnormalities

However, taking this medication may result in oily hair and skin. It is also important to remember that there is still controversy regarding treatment with DHEA with some authorities still not convinced of its effectiveness and regard it as experimental. It is always worth seeking advice from your fertility clinic/doctor before taking this supplement.

What are the author's views on DHEA?

After looking at the evidence for the use of DHEA, although not absolute, there does seem to be some evidence for its use. However, I would not use it as a first line and I would not use it if I had responded adequately to the IVF drugs. I would, however, think about using DHEA for 3 months prior to an IVF cycle *IF* I had had a previous poor response in previous cycles.

Where can I get DHEA from?

Micronized DHEA can be obtained with a prescription from a pharmacy. Ask your fertility unit to advise you on this.

Co-Enzyme Q10

Co-Enzyme Q10 or Ubiquinone is a substance that naturally occurs within the body, that appears to diminish in concentration the older we get. Its function is to help generate energy within the cells of the body. The human egg is a large cell that when penetrated by a sperm has lots of little "factories" (the biological name for these factories is Mitochondria) that produce lots of energy to drive the development of a normal embryo. One **theory** is that the older the egg, the less Co-Enzyme Q10 these little factories contain, and so the less energy the fertilised egg can produce to drive the development of a normal healthy embryo. Supplementation of the diet with Co-Enzyme Q10 may **theoretically** enhance the performance of these little factories within the egg to improve energy production and hence provide a positive effect on the genetic material within the fertilised egg to improve egg quality and implantation.

Co-Enzyme Q10 is not a prescription medication, and can be bought over the counter. It is being used by a number of older women undergoing IVF to theoretically improve their egg quality. More scientific research needs to be done to determine if it is really helpful in improving egg quality – but there is no evidence to date that it does any harm if taken before an IVF cycle in doses of 200mg daily.

Testosterone/Testosterone Patches

There is some evidence that the use of testosterone gel applied to the skin (transdermal) can increase in the live birth rate in IVF patients who were previously found to be poor responders if used 3-4 weeks before the start of IVF cycle. Again I would not use testosterone *unless* I had had a poor response in previous IVF cycles. Discussion with your IVF doctor is warranted about its use in the event that you do not respond to the medication to stimulate your ovaries.

Steroids

Steroids are widely used in Medicine to treat inflammatory conditions – so for example, if you have eczema – steroid cream (Hydrocortisone) is used, if you have asthma – steroid inhalers are used. In some patients the production of antibodies against their own body parts can cause an inflammatory response that can affect their fertility. For example, some women may produce antibodies against their own ovaries (anti-ovarian-antibodies) or against their thyroid gland (anti-thyroid antibodies). There is some evidence that the use of steroids in such cases when women have previously responded poorly to IVF treatment may be beneficial. In addition, there is no evidence that low dose steroid tablets (for example Prednisolone 5mg) does any harm.

What are the author's views on steroids?

In the event of a patient having previous failed cycles, in addition to an inflammatory condition with circulating antibodies against her ovaries or thyroid gland or others – I would certainly consider the use of a small dose of steroid during a subsequent cycle.

Aspirin

Aspirin seems to be the "cure all" for a great many conditions. For example there is evidence that it acts to reduce the risk of bowel cancer, reduce the risk of strokes, reduce the risk of a repeat heart attack, and reduce the risk of thrombosis (formation of blood clots). It acts by reducing inflammation as well as being a "blood thinner". Some authorities feel that because it acts as a blood thinner it may improve the blood supply to the ovaries and improve ovarian response in IVF treatment. There is however, NO good evidence that Aspirin can improve your chances when undergoing IVF. In fact there is some evidence that Aspirin can actually reduce your chances of ovulation, implantation, and increase your risk of spontaneous miscarriage.

However, if you suffer from **Recurrent Miscarriage Syndrome** (defined as three miscarriages in a row) AND you suffer from a condition called Anti-phospholipid Syndrome (see chapter 8 on miscarriage), then once pregnant, there is some evidence that Aspirin can help improve your chance of successful outcome of a live birth.

If given, Aspirin is usually given as a low dose tablet of 75mg daily. It is available over the counter and does not need a prescription. However, I would seek advice from your clinic or doctor before using it. There are side effects including allergic reactions, upset stomach, heartburn – although if used in a low dose (75mg), side effects are usually minimal.

What are the author's views on Aspirin?

Generally, I would not use Aspirin in women undergoing an IVF cycle. Furthermore, I would not use Aspirin in early pregnancy since there is some evidence that it can increase the risk of miscarriage in the early stages, UNLESS I had a diagnosis of Recurrent Miscarriage Syndrome (3 consecutive miscarriages) and had Anti-phospholipid Syndrome.

Clexane (Low molecular weight Heparin)

Clexane is a substance that essentially "thins" the blood and makes it less "sticky". It is a small injection usually given on a daily basis. In mainstream medicine, it is used to prevent and to treat thrombosis (formation of blood clots). It is safe to use in pregnancy. There is some evidence that in women who have a tendency to develop blood clots (the scientific name for this is thrombophilia), and in women with Recurrent Miscarriage Syndrome (with a condition called Anti-phospholipid Syndrome), *Clexane* can be beneficial in improving live birth rates if given from the day of embryo transfer until birth. The usual dose in *Clexane* 40mg injected daily.

It is also interesting that *Clexane* has a role in modifying the immune system and preliminary studies have suggested that it might be useful when used with steroids in patients undergoing IVF, particularly if there is a history "inflammatory conditions".

What are the author's views on *Clexane*?

In patients with a history of recurrent miscarriage or a tendency to form blood clots (thrombophilia), the use of *Clexane* makes absolute sense and I have a LOW threshold for the use of *Clexane* following IVF and throughout pregnancy. Side effects include irritation at the site of injection, thinning of the bones (osteoporosis) after prolonged use, hair loss (very rarely), and reduction of platelets (a component of the blood that helps with formation of blood clots). This last side effect is very rare and I have never seen it in patients that I have treated. Periodic blood tests to check the platelets is sensible. Some doctors recommend the use of calcium tablets (500mg twice per day) to help prevent bone thinning if *Clexane* is taken for prolonged periods of time.

For Him – *Condensyl*

There may be known or unknown harm to sperm caused by "Oxidative Damage". This is damage to the DNA of the sperm by environmental pollution (e.g. traffic fumes, toxins in heavy industry, cigarette smoking) and environmental radiation. It therefore makes sense to include "anti-oxidants" in your diet to combat this and potentially improve the quality of your sperm. A new tablet was recently launched called *Condensyl*. This appears to boost the body's natural anti-oxidant defence and subsequently may achieve a better pregnancy rate. Clinical studies thus far have indicated an improvement in pregnancy rates in couples who had previously been resistant to IVF and ICSI. It is thought that the use of *Condensyl* may also help in achieving natural conception in couples who have been struggling. Since men produce a new batch of sperm every 3-4 months, the advice is that you need to take the *Condensyl* daily for 4 months to achieve the best sperm result.

What are the author's views on *Condensyl*?

There does appear to be some evidence that this is beneficial, and as such I would be inclined to use it both in patients struggling with natural conception or indeed in patients undergoing IVF / ICSI.

Condensyl can be obtained from the internet (https://condensyl.co.uk/condensyl-from-pharmasure)

Embryological Factors

The Embryoscope

This is a cutting-edge embryo incubator that essentially employs time lapse photography to film the progress of the developing embryos. A photograph is taken every 15 minutes so that development of each embryo from the time of fertilisation to the time of embryo transfer is recorded. Hence, when each embryo is ready to be placed back into the womb not only can the embryo be graded according to what it looks like now, but also the development of each embryo from the earliest stages can be assessed. If there has been abnormal development noted by reviewing images from the Embryoscope, then that embryo is less likely to produce a viable pregnancy. On the other hand if the embryo has shown normal development as witnessed by the Embryoscope, then it is more likely to yield a viable pregnancy. In this way the Embryoscope provides more information on how to choose the best embryos for embryo transfer to improve the chance of a positive pregnancy test and ongoing pregnancy.

Assisted Hatching

Around each embryo is a shell just like the chick in a bird's egg. Just as the chick needs to hatch out of its shell, so too does the human embryo need to hatch out of its own shell in order to implant into the lining of the womb. It is thought that one of the reasons that there is failure of implantation of the embryo is because that embryo has failed to hatch out of its shell. This is easily remedied by a procedure called "Assisted Hatching". This is carried out by a qualified embryologist who essentially holds the embryo and with the use of fine laser makes a tiny hole within the shell of the embryo prior to embryo transfer, which facilitates hatching. In the right hands, there is very little risk to the embryo, although the risk of identical twins is increased by a tiny amount (about 1%). Assisted Hatching is usually recommended if the female partner is more than 40 years of age, if the embryologist thinks the egg shell looks particularly thick, and finally if there is a history of failed implantation in previous cycles.

Embryo Glue

This is a great marketing name, but is certainly nothing like glue. The embryos can be placed into "Embryo Glue" prior to their transfer into the womb. It is thought this facilitates communication between cells and is helpful for the process of implantation. Some embryologists feel that there is a small advantage to using this prior to embryo transfer.

IMSI

IMSI stands for **Intracytoplasmic Morphological Sperm Injection**. In English, this means that when the embryologist is looking for the best single sperm to use for injection, they use a special microscope that is x6000 more powerful to assess each sperm. In this way tiny defects in the sperm that would not ordinarily have been seen are detected and only "perfect" sperm used to inject into the egg. Hence IMSI is a useful selection tool for the embryologist in choosing the best sperm. IMSI is recommended in couples in whom there is recurrent implantation failure, failed ICSI or indeed in sperm samples with many of the sperm showing an abnormal form or shape.

PGS

PGS stands for **Pre-implantation Genetic Screening** and is a process that occurs in IVF or ICSI cycles after the egg collection and formation of any embryo(s). From each embryo a cell or cells are taken and examined for genetic (chromosomal) abnormalities. Thereafter, only the good embryo(s) – or those without genetic (chromosomal) abnormalities are replaced back into the uterus. The procedure is intended to improve pregnancy success rates and reduce miscarriage rates, however to date, there is little evidence to show that PGS improves success rates in older women or those with recurrent miscarriage. Although, interestingly there is some evidence that it improves success rates in women less than 37 years old with no history of miscarriage.

There is more information on this from the HFEA website (www.hfea.gov.uk).

What are the author's views on these Embryological Factors?

I would certainly recommend the use of the first four of these procedures, but since there is no good evidence to date that PGS is effective in improving success rates in IVF / ICSI cycles particularly for women with a history of previous failed cycles or those with a history of recurrent miscarriage, I would be disinclined to recommend it. Furthermore it is not available on the NHS, and if IVF is undertaken in a private clinic it is rather expensive.

Acupuncture

The use of acupuncture in improving IVF outcomes is

debatable and unproven. Generally there is no good scientific evidence for its use that I can find in the scientific literature. However, I am aware that anecdotally, a number of women find it useful and certainly there is no evidence that it does any harm.

Pre-existing Medical Complaints

It is important any pre-existing medical or surgical condition is reviewed before embarking on a pregnancy. This is important for a number of reasons. The first is that poor control of certain medical conditions can have a very real adverse effect on the proposed pregnancy. Poorly controlled diabetes can increase congenital abnormalities and miscarriage. There is an association with abnormal thyroid function and miscarriage/infertility. Epilepsy and in particular the drugs used to treat it can have a deleterious effect on the pregnancy. Drugs used to treat depression can have an effect on the development of a baby's heart. Drugs used for all sorts of other medical conditions can have an adverse effect on not only your chances of a successful IVF cycle, but also your chances of a successful ongoing trouble free pregnancy. So the message is, seek medical help to effectively treat whatever the condition that you have is, and ensure that the medication used to treat it is pregnancy friendly.

Lifestyle Factors

Obesity – carrying excess weight correlates with menstrual cycle disturbance and infertility. Weight loss of just 5% can result in restoration of ovulation in women with deranged menstrual cycles. The advantages of maintaining a healthy weight are obvious.

Alcohol – excess alcohol can lead to disorders of ovulation and even stop a woman having periods altogether. Alcohol consumed in early pregnancy can lead to physical malformations, intellectual disability, and growth restriction. There is some evidence that if you stop drinking alcohol completely you improve your fertility. In IVF cycles, consumption of alcohol was associated with reduction in pregnancy rates and increased miscarriage rates. It is also interesting that consumption of alcohol in the male partner was also associated with a reduction in achieving an ongoing pregnancy.

Smoking – there is evidence that smoking reduces ovarian reserve (kills off eggs), reduces the chances of getting pregnant, and reduces the chances of a fertility treatment being successful. Moreover, smoking during pregnancy increases the risk of miscarriage, increases the risk of pre-term labour, increases the risk of growth restriction of the baby – this is easy – DO NOT SMOKE.

Statistics
It is important to remember that statistics play a major role in successful IVF/ICSI outcome. In the best hands and optimum conditions (young age, good AMH, no medical or surgical problems), pregnancy rates of 50-60% are seen, with "take home baby" rates of about 30-40% per cycle. This means that more couples are disappointed following an IVF cycle than are elated. Find out what the expectations for your age group are and be realistic about your chances. Sometimes the best thing you can do is to be persistent and have another cycle. However, this needs to be put into context – I would not advise this in a 43-year-old woman who has an approximate 5% chance of a successful outcome in any IVF cycle using her own eggs. **A**

lot of the time, the answer is in the age of the woman and
more precisely her eggs. Hence the paragraph below on the
use of donor eggs.

Use of Donor Eggs

Probably the single most important factor in determining the
success of any IVF procedure is a determinant that the couple
can do nothing about – maternal age, or more specifically the
age of the eggs. As already stated, many women leave it too
late to start their family. After 35 years of age, a woman's fertility significantly reduces and her miscarriage rate significantly
increases. IVF appears to be more successful at achieving
pregnancy per cycle than natural means, yet at the age of 43,
a woman has approximately a 5% chance of having a baby
with IVF. That means she is going through a procedure that is
costing her emotionally, physically, and financially with a 95%
chance that it will not work. Furthermore, if she is more than
45 years of age she has an approximate 93% chance of miscarriage. So what is to be done to help that couple achieve the
dream of having their own child? The answer is to use donor
eggs. Utilising the eggs of a young woman fertilised by your
partner's sperm is much more likely to give rise to a successful outcome. There are a number of factors I often quote to
couples when they are deciding on whether to use donor eggs.

How similar is the genetic material between my eggs and those of a would-be donor?

The answer is that 99.5% of the genetic material between 2
human beings is the same. So when a couple state that donor
eggs are not the same as their own they are right, but only 0.5%
right – the rest of the genetic material is the same.

Can the embryo derived from a donor egg and growing in me be affected by the environment of my womb?

The answer to this question is absolutely yes. The growing embryo is influenced by your hormones, your blood supply to the uterus, your nutrition, and the environment in which the embryo grows. The pregnant woman shapes and determines the baby's future which carries 99.5% of her genetic material in any case.

Is the baby conceived by a donor egg really the recipient's baby?

The embryo already has 99.5% of his or her mother's genetic material. The embryo grows within that mother's womb, under the influence of her hormones, nutrition, blood supply, feelings, thoughts, and dare I say it, love. The mother then goes through labour and gives birth to deliver her baby. Is this her baby? I think so.

So the message is:

1. If you have a pre-existing medical or surgical condition, it needs to be optimised. For example, if you are diabetic, good control before pregnancy can have a massive effect on reduction of miscarriage and congenital abnormality. Likewise pre-pregnancy review of other medical conditions is a must.

2. Alter lifestyle factors. Avoid smoking, drinking alcohol, and aim for a normal body weight.

3. Be aware of the success rates of IVF according to your age and AMH, if you are an older woman consider the use of donor eggs. Remember that donor eggs carry 99.5% of your own genetic material.

4. If you have had a previous failed implantation in an IVF cycle, consider an Endometrial Scratch.
5. If you have a history of recurrent miscarriage or have an inflammatory condition, consider the use of a small dose *Clexane*/steroids.
6. If you are older, and have a history of poor response to medication given to stimulate your ovaries, consider using DHEA/Testosterone gel.
7. Remember IVF is a statistics game, ask your chance of success and plan accordingly.
8. If there was any one magical factor that made a huge difference to IVF success rates – everyone would use it. That having been said *it is* worth considering some off licence* options that may help to promote success rates.

*In the UK, prescribed medicines have a license to be used for particular conditions or illnesses. If a medication is used "Off-licence" it means it is being prescribed in an unusual and unlicensed way. Some medications utilised in the hope that they will improve IVF outcome (DHEA, Steroids, Testosterone, *Clexane*) are often used anecdotally and off-license. It is advisable to check with your GP or fertility doctor before using them.

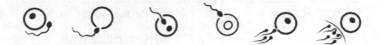

CHAPTER 8

Miscarriage

How common is miscarriage?

Overall 15-20% of pregnancies end in miscarriage. That means up to every 5th woman you see on the street has miscarried.

Miscarriage is a cruel and heartbreaking phenomenon, but is massively common in the general population. The older the woman becomes, the more common it is. You will remember that unlike men who make new batches of sperm every 3 months, a woman is born with a finite number of eggs and these age as the woman gets older, so that by the time the woman gets into her 40s her miscarriage rate goes up beyond 30%.

Again, the message is:
    "If at all possible have your children before you reach 40 years of age."

Age Range	Approximate Miscarriage Rate
Up to 19 years old	12% to 14%
20-24 years old	10% to 12%
25-29 years old	11% to 13%
30-34 years old	14% to 16%
35-39 years old	24% to 26%
40-44 years old	>50%
>45 years old	>90%

When I see couples who have been through a miscarriage, the vast majority of women will feel that they have done something to cause the loss of their baby. They blame themselves for this natural phenomenon. "If only I hadn't had that single glass of wine, done that shopping, lifted that object, gone for that long walk." The list is endless as they try to make sense of their loss. But the truth is that early pregnancy is an all or nothing event. Generally, if it is going to happen, there is very little that you can do to prevent it and nothing that you have done to cause it. The vast majority of miscarriages (up to 60%) are because of DNA or chromosomal abnormalities in the developing foetus or baby. The older you are, the greater the risk. For example, a woman's age-related risk of having a baby with Down's syndrome is 1 in 1,000 when she is 30 years old, but it is 1 in 100 when she is 40 years old – a tenfold increase. Some couples will take a small amount of solace from the fact that although miscarriage is a very distressing time, sometimes miscarriage is kinder than the eventual birth of a deformed or genetically abnormal baby. So please remember:

'There is nothing that you have done to cause the miscarriage and certainly because it is very common for the woman especially to blame herself – please be reassured – you have not caused it. It is not your fault.'

As an aside I will also mention that although the age of the potential father is not as important as the age of the potential mother, it is thought that once the man's age goes beyond 40 years old the risk of miscarriage starts to go up.

If I have miscarried once already, what is my risk of miscarrying in my next pregnancy?
It is important to know, however, that if a woman (less than 35 years of age) has 1 miscarriage, her risk of miscarrying in the next, second pregnancy is still of the order of 15-20%.

If I have miscarried twice in a row, what is my risk of miscarriage in my next pregnancy?
If the same woman miscarries the second pregnancy, then her chance of miscarriage for the third pregnancy still remains about the same (15-20%).

If I have miscarried three times in a row, what is my risk of miscarriage in my next pregnancy?
When a woman has miscarried 3 times in a row she has a diagnosis of **Recurrent Miscarriage Syndrome (RSM)**, and now

the chance of a future pregnancy miscarrying is of the order of 40%. Hence, RMS is defined as 3 miscarriages consecutively and is a syndrome present in 1% of the female population. This needs to be medically investigated.

It is important to state that the 40% risk of miscarriage is only present if there have been 3 consecutive miscarriages. If for example you have had 2 miscarriages followed by a normal pregnancy with delivery of a healthy child, and thereafter suffer from another miscarriage – this is not recurrent miscarriage syndrome. It has to be 3 consecutive miscarriages one after the after.

What are the causes of miscarriage?
As already discussed, the majority of miscarriages (up to 60%) are because of DNA or chromosomal abnormalities in the developing foetus or baby, and the older you are the greater the risk. This does not mean that the pregnant woman or her partner have abnormal chromosomes, it is merely when the egg and sperm get together there is a mismatch of genetic material and the chance of this happening increases with the increasing age of the egg. To confirm that this has occurred you can ask for the products of conception passed during miscarriage to be sent off for genetic analysis.

When a miscarriage occurs three times in a row then as already stated the diagnosis is that of Recurrent Miscarriage Syndrome and investigations need to be carried out. There is no reason why your GP cannot do this for you. Hence the causes of RMS are as follows:

i.   **Antiphospholipid Syndrome** – this is a posh name for a condition that occurs in approximately 15% of women with RMS and is important because it is *treatable*.

A blood test specifically looking for this can be done by your doctor. Left untreated the chance of a live birth is only about 10%. With treatment, the miscarriage rate is reduced by up to 50-60%.

ii. **Genetic/chromosomal rearrangements of the parents** – this occurs in approximately 4% of couples with recurrent miscarriage. If the genetic testing of the products of conception show a particular sort of chromosomal abnormality then testing of the parents is carried out. This, again, is a blood test.

iii. **Congenital abnormalities of the womb** – some women have a split or partitioned womb, others half a womb and so on. This is unusual and is usually identified with an ultrasound scan.

iv. **Weakness of the cervix or neck of the womb** – this usually manifests itself because the miscarriage occurs in the second trimester (between week 12 and week 24 of the pregnancy) after the neck of the womb in essence opens up with loss of the baby.

v. **Hormone factors** – this can be divided into 3 main categories:

   a. The first is diabetes. Uncontrolled diabetes with high sugar levels is associated with miscarriage and foetal abnormalities. However, once identified and treated, the trend for miscarriage and foetal abnormalities is reversed. A simple blood test (HbA1c) carried out on the mother can look for this.

   b. The second is thyroid disease. An overactive thyroid gland gives rise to symptoms of diarrhoea and weight loss. An underactive thyroid gland gives rise to symptoms of being cold, tired, and constipated.

Both under and overactive thyroid disease can result in miscarriage. A simple blood test (TFTs – Thyroid Function Tests) can be carried out. Treatment of thyroid disease can reduce the risk of miscarriage.

c. Polycystic Ovarian Syndrome. This can lead to a "diabetic-like" state which is thought by some to increase the risk of miscarriage. Therefore the anti-diabetic medication Metformin has been used to treat women with PCOS who have had recurrent miscarriage, although the evidence that this helps is limited. However, there is no evidence that Metformin does any harm in pregnancy.

vi. **Immune Factors** – there is much talk of "Natural Killer" (NK) cells that exist in the bloodstream and in the uterus (endometrial lining) that may affect pregnancy and abnormalities of these may cause miscarriage. This is very much research based at present. Abnormal NK cells in the blood stream are not thought to have any effect on miscarriage, however there is a link between abnormal NK cells in the endometrial lining of the womb and miscarriage. The use of steroids (for example *Prednisolone*) has been shown to reduce the numbers of abnormal NK cells in the endometrial lining but has not been associated with any reduction in miscarriage rates. Despite this, some doctors recommend a small dose of steroid in women who have had recurrent miscarriage. Routine testing for these factors is not recommended by the Royal College of Obstetricians and Gynaecologists in their latest guideline.

vii. **Infection** – A one-off bad infection can cause miscarriage, but it is not thought to be the cause of recurrent miscarriage since you would have to consistently have repeated bad infections (flu-like symptoms) every time you had a pregnancy. However, there is some evidence that "Bacterial Vaginosis" has been linked to miscarriage both early and later on in the pregnancy. One study showed that the use of a particular antibiotic (Clindamycin) used after 12 weeks of pregnancy reduced the risk of subsequent miscarriage and preterm birth.

viii. **Inherited clotting defects (Thrombophilia screen)** – There is a list of blood tests that can be done looking at whether a woman with recurrent miscarriage has abnormalities with blood that tends to clot excessively. These include – Factor V Leiden, Prothrombin Gene Variant, Protein C and S deficiency, Hyperhomocystenaemia and antithrombin III. Various studies have shown that these abnormalities may be associated with an increased frequency of recurrent miscarriage and in particular late miscarriage. These defects which are associated with an increased tendency to cause blood clots, can be treated to prevent blood clots in pregnancy and there is some evidence that treatment can reduce miscarriage rates.

So what should I do? My feelings on the matter and generally what happens in real life:

After 1 miscarriage

I wouldn't be inclined to have any tests. Miscarriage is so common that starting a battery of tests after 1 single miscarriage would not be appropriate. I would simply get on with the process of getting pregnant again. The fact that you got pregnant in the first place is reassuring.

After 2 consecutive miscarriages

Some couples ask to be investigated at this point for fear of the third pregnancy miscarrying, which could have been avoided if investigations and then treatment for any abnormalities had been carried out. I have some sympathy with this chain of thought, particularly if the woman is 35 years old or more when her miscarriage rate is starting to go up anyway and her fertility is starting to reduce. The tests at this point would be the same as for 3 consecutive miscarriages.

After 3 consecutive miscarriages

You need investigation and I would do the following investigations:

i.   Antiphospholipid screening – blood test
ii. Thyroid Function test and HBA1c (test for diabetes) – both blood tests
iii. Ultrasound scan of the pelvis to ensure normal anatomy
iv. Ensure genetic testing of "products of conception" (tissue from your womb following the miscarriage). If this was abnormal then chromosomal analysis of both partners – blood tests for the woman and her partner is required.
v.   Thrombophilia screen – blood test to see if clotting is normal, particularly if one of the miscarriages occurred later than 10 weeks.

In addition, if a late miscarriage (greater than 12 weeks) previously occurred:

i.   I would take a vaginal swab when the pregnancy is 10-12 weeks gestation, to identify "bacterial vaginosis" and if this is present, I would be treat it with antibiotics.

ii. I would carry out serial ultrasound scans of the cervical length (length of the neck of the womb) every 1-2 weeks and if this shortens to less than 2.5cm I would discuss the insertion of a stitch in the neck of the womb with the couple.

iii. I would not be inclined to have immune testing and the Royal College of Obstetricians and Gynaecologists guidelines agree with this.

So now what treatment is sensible?

1. Regular follow-up and ultrasound scans are reassuring and may help during the course of early pregnancy.

2. If diabetes is picked up, then good control can minimise your risk of miscarriage and future congenital abnormalities.

3. If thyroid disease is identified, treatment with thyroxine is thought to reduce miscarriage rates.

4. If Antiphospholipid screening is positive, then treatment with low dose aspirin (75mg daily) and a small injection of enoxaparin 40mg daily (otherwise known as *Clexane*) from conception onwards is thought to be beneficial. *Clexane* is commonly known as a "blood thinner" and reduces the incidence of blood clots.

5. If genetic abnormalities are present, then referral to a specialist genetic counsellor is appropriate.

6. There is some evidence that progesterone use in early pregnancy either as pessaries (commonly known as *Cyclogest or Utrogestin*) or injections (*Gestone*) can help – they do no harm so I use them.

7. If the "thrombophilia screen" (abnormal blood clotting tests) is positive, women can be at risk of thrombosis

(clots commonly in the legs and even lungs). Since there is also some evidence that a positive thrombophilia screen is associated with miscarriage, it does not seem unreasonable to use *Clexane* 40mg daily in these women.

8. Some doctors use a small dose of steroid (usually pred-nisolone 5-10mg) in early pregnancy because the theory is that if there is an immunity problem in terms of the pregnant patient's body attacking the pregnancy to cause recurrent miscarriage, then a steroid should reduce that attack, and in doing so theoretically reduce the chance of miscarriage. There is no overwhelming evidence to support this, however, and careful discussion with your doctor is advised.

9. If there is a congenital abnormality of the womb, (for example some women have a partition or "septum" dividing the womb in half), some doctors would rec-ommend surgery to remove the septum or partition. It is thought that approximately 65-85% of patients with this physical abnormality of their womb will have a suc-cessful pregnancy after surgery to remove the septum. However, approximately 60% of the same group of women will have a successful pregnancy without sur-gery and if they continue to try and get pregnant up to around 80% of them will eventually have a live baby. Therefore careful discussion with your doctor is needed. Surgery has its own risks and it is not yet proven to be the best thing to do.

So what happens if you have recurrent miscarriage but ALL the tests are normal?

It is not uncommon to have all these tests carried out and

they are all normal. If this is the case, the good news is that approximately 75% of the time the next pregnancy will be successful with supportive care alone (in other words regular medical follow-up/ultrasound scans/reassurance). This percentage of course goes down with increasing age, particularly of the mother.

Even if all the tests are negative, many doctors will treat the woman in early pregnancy with the following:

i. Progesterone pessaries or injections – These help to stabilise the lining of the womb (endometrium) and the theory is that they help to prevent the lining of the womb (to which the developing foetus is attached) from coming away. The evidence for this is limited, but certainly there is no evidence that it does any harm.

ii. Aspirin – For many years some doctors have encouraged the use of low dose Aspirin (75mg daily) in women who have had miscarriages. There is evidence that it is useful in women with recurrent miscarriage who have been diagnosed with antiphospholipid syndrome and in women who have suffered with toxaemia (pre-eclampsia) in a previous pregnancy. However, in women with unexplained recurrent miscarriage syndrome, recent evidence has suggested that Aspirin may actually increase the risk of miscarriage in early pregnancy if taken in the first 12 weeks. Therefore, if all your tests are negative, it would seem sensible not to take Aspirin, at least not in the first 12 weeks of pregnancy.

iii. Enoxaparin (*Clexane*) – *Clexane* can very rarely cause thinning of the bones and something called "thrombocytopenia", which in English means it reduces the numbers of tiny little particles in the bloodstream called platelets. These help with the clotting process. This is very rare and the vast, vast number of women on *Clexane* will have no problems. Some doctors prescribe *Clexane* for women with unexplained Recurrent Miscarriage Syndrome because it is unlikely to cause any harm, and it *may* help. There may be some clotting or immune factor in recurrent miscarriage syndrome that the scientific community is not even aware of, a factor that might be treated with *Clexane*.

iv. Steroids – To reiterate, some doctors prescribe Steroids for women with unexplained Recurrent Miscarriage Syndrome because it is unlikely to cause any harm, and it may help. There may be some immune factor in recurrent miscarriage syndrome that the scientific community is not even aware of, a factor that might be treated with a small dose of steroid, such as Prednisolone 5mg daily. This may be particularly relevant in woman who suffer with an inflammatory / immune condition.

A Clinical Story

Mrs X was a young married woman with no children. She had been trying to have a baby for many years and had suffered with no less than 5 miscarriages one after the other. She had been thoroughly reviewed and tested by experts in Recurrent Miscarriage Syndrome and told that there were no reasons that they could find regarding the cause of her miscarriages. She was advised that no treatment was necessary but to just continue to try and have children.

When she was subsequently seen in the very early stages of her sixth pregnancy, she was distraught at the thought of what was to come. She and her partner felt that they had nothing to lose and asked for empirical treatment with *Clexane*, a small dose of steroid (*Prednisolone* 5mg), progesterone pessaries (*Cyclogest*), and regular support in the form of ultrasound scans and clinical follow-up. This treatment was initiated at the couple's request and they were made aware that there was no overwhelming evidence for its use.

Mrs X got to 39 weeks gestation before delivering a healthy and much longed-for baby. Eighteen months later the couple found themselves pregnant again and the same medication package was instituted with the same joyous result.

To this day I do not know if the treatment given to this couple influenced the outcome, but it certainly appeared to be more than just coincidence that after 5 disasters, treatment was given with the resulting 2 bundles of joy.

So the main messages:
1. Do not wait too long to have your children, the risk of miscarriage goes up with increasing age, especially after 35 years of age.
2. Do not wait too long to have your children, the risk of chromosomal abnormality (for example, Down's syndrome) goes up with increasing age.
3. If you are young and have had 3 miscarriages in a row, you NEED investigation – do not be fobbed off.
4. If you are older, and have had 2 miscarriages in a row, it may not be unreasonable to ask for investigations.
5. Find an empathetic, supportive doctor or clinic. Empirical treatment as above is not unreasonable for patients who feel that they have nothing to lose.

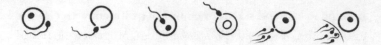

CHAPTER 9A

Polycystic Ovarian Syndrome (PCOS)

What is Polycystic Ovarian Syndrome (PCOS)?

This is a condition commonly seen in women who do not have regular periods and who do not ovulate (release an egg) on a regular basis. Hence it is frequently seen in women presenting with infertility. It is the commonest hormonal condition affecting women of child bearing age, occurring in 5 to 10% of that population so, if you have PCOS, there are many others like you. The phrase "polycystic" is an inappropriate name for this condition because the ovaries do not contain "cysts" in the true sense of the word, they merely contain follicles that have stopped growing. A better name would be "Poly-follicular Ovarian Syndrome". The follicles are usually no more than 9mm in diameter, in other words hardly "cystic" (a good going ovarian cyst is 5cm or more) and despite what women are often told, these "Poly-follicular" ovaries do NOT give rise to pain.

The definition of PCOS (according to the European Society of Human Reproduction and Embryology) includes 2 out of 3 criteria:

  i.   Infrequent periods (irregular or prolonged times between periods) or anovulation (no ovulation).

ii.   Physical signs of excessive androgens (testosterone) like excessive hair growth/acne or blood tests indicating excessive androgens (testosterone).

iii. Ultrasound scan evidence of polycystic ovaries.

From the above, you can therefore see that if a woman has polycystic ovaries on ultrasound, but has regular periods and no evidence of excessive hair growth/acne, she does NOT have Polycystic Ovarian *Syndrome* because she only has 1 out of 3 criteria. Women can have polycystic ovaries on ultrasound scan and regularly ovulate.

Are women with polycystic ovaries obese? Does losing weight help to improve their fertility?

It is thought that about 40-50% of PCOS women are obese, so conversely many women with PCOS are relatively slim. This means there is great variability in how PCOS presents. Patients with PCOS may be obese or slim, have problems with excess body hair or not, have problems with acne or have clear skin, may have polycystic ovaries on ultrasound or may not. It is the combination of factors as above that leads to the diagnosis.

It is upsetting for women with PCOS who are obese, that further weight gain can worsen established symptoms of excessive body hair, acne, and irregular periods with reduced chances of ovulation. **Weight loss, on the other hand**, is likely to reduce symptoms of acne, excess body hair, whilst promoting regular periods and even ovulation.

What happens to the hormones in PCOS?

When ordering blood tests, your doctor should include:

i.   Testosterone – levels of this go up in PCOS and this is what causes the increase in body and facial hair together with acne.

ii.   LH – Luteinising Hormone – the level of LH goes up in PCOS in comparison to the level of FSH – Follicle Stimulating Hormone. You will remember from previous chapters that it is the LH surge that is responsible for ovulation. But if the LH is continuously raised there is no surge and there is no ovulation. Therefore be careful interpreting LH ovulation kits that you buy over the counter since a high level of LH may not mean that you have ovulated that month.

iii. Oestrogen – levels of this hormone are the same or higher in PCOS. Oestrogen causes growth of the lining of the womb (endometrium) in preparation for the embryo to implant.

iv.   Progesterone – you will remember from previous chapters that progesterone is produced by the ovarian follicle that has released an egg and collapses becoming a "corpus luteum". Progesterone stabilises the lining of the womb that has previously grown under the influence of oestrogen. If it is stopped or withdrawn, then the endometrium no longer is stabilised and breaks down, causing you to have a period. In PCOS, there is no ovulation, hence there is no collapsed follicle or "corpus luteum", hence there is no progesterone production, hence there is no eventual progesterone withdrawal, hence women do have regular breakdown of the lining of the womb or periods. This means that the lining of the womb can continue to grow under the influence of oestrogen, which can lead to thickened and abnormal changes in the endometrial lining.

v.   AMH – this is usually very high in patients with PCOS. This means that there are plenty of eggs in the ovaries of patients with PCOS, but they are not being released.

How do you test to see if you are ovulating?
See Chapter 4 (So what investigations do you need?).

How do you treat women with PCOS who are not ovulating?
In women with established PCOS, and indeed in women who are not getting pregnant because they are not ovulating, a medication called "*Clomid or Clomifene*" is often used. *Clomid* works by interacting with a part of the human brain (the hypothalamus and pituitary gland) to produce a surge of FSH (Follicle Stimulating Hormone) that in turn stimulates the ovaries to develop follicles with eggs in them.

Clomid is essentially a tablet that comes in 50mg, 100mg, or 150mg strengths. If day 1 of a woman's cycle is when she starts her period, then initially *Clomid* 50mg is taken starting on day 2 and continuing to day 6 (5 days in total during that cycle). This will usually result in a woman ovulating around day 14, hence giving her a 28 day cycle.

To ensure ovulation has occurred, a Day 21 Progesterone level blood test (as above) can be taken to ensure the level is >30mmol/l (if the Progesterone blood test shows >30mmol, the ovulation is likely to have occurred). Alternatively, follicle tracking can be carried out with regular ultrasound scans to image the developing follicle(s) and the resultant corpus luteum(s) confirming ovulation has taken place. If ovulation has not occurred, then the dose of *Clomid* is increased to 100mg during the course of the next cycle. The risks of taking *Clomid* include multiple pregnancy (twins ~10-15% / triplets ~1%) and because the ovaries are being pushed to produce follicles then the risk of cystic change in the ovaries goes up. About 10% of women will experience hot flushes.

Finally, if you are not having any periods it is difficult to start *Clomid* on day 2 because you haven't had a period! The answer is to use a progesterone. So if you have not had a period for 2 months or longer, then check a pregnancy test to make sure that you are pregnant. If this is negative, then start a progesterone tablet, such as Norethisterone (5mg) three times daily for 5 days. You will remember that progesterone stabilises the lining of the womb (endometrium) so that when it is stopped after 5 days, the endometrium is destabilised and menstruation starts. Count this as day 1, then the following day (day 2) start *Clomid*.

So what are the success rates and what other treatments are available if *Clomid* doesn't work?

About 70% of the time, *Clomid* helps non-ovulatory women to produce an egg and if all else is normal with the couple, then up to 50% of couples will have achieved pregnancy within 6 months. Many doctors will use *Clomid* for up to 9 months, if it has not worked by then other options include:

i.   The use of Gonadotrophin injections like FSH as in IUI/IVF cycles to stimulate the ovaries to produce follicles that produce eggs.

ii.   The use of *Metformin* – although studies suggest that this is less successful at inducing ovulation compared to *Clomid*. However, it may help in reducing weight in obese patients with PCOS as well as improving your chance of ovulating.

iii. Laparoscopic Ovarian Drilling – this is essentially key-hole surgery that then burns little holes in the ovary or ovaries. The way this works is unknown, but it does seem to help with cycle control and stimulate ovulation particularly in patients with high LH levels.

iv. If ovulation does not occur with 100mg *Clomid,* there is no evidence that increasing the dose to 150mg is beneficial.

Finally, there is no justification in using Clomid in someone who is already be shown to be ovulating. This may even reduce your chance of becoming pregnant.

Extras you need to know about PCOS

i. Women with PCOS have something called increased insulin resistance, which means that they are more likely to become diabetic. It is also true that women with PCOS are much more likely to become diabetic (Type 2 non-insulin dependent diabetes) in comparison to other women in the general population. Therefore, it is even more important to watch their diet and exercise regularly. Plenty of exercise, a healthy diet, and avoidance of obesity is likely to reverse this trend in middle age.

ii. Obese patients with PCOS have an increase in the risk of "Obstructive sleep apnoea". In English this means that they are more likely to snore at night and have fatigue and sleepiness during the day. This in itself may contribute to insulin resistance and effect that woman's quality of life. There is effective treatment for this – so see your GP..

iii. In the event that you become pregnant, you must have a

"Glucose Tolerance Test" (GTT) at around 28 weeks of the pregnancy. This is because you are much more likely to get "gestational diabetes" which makes the pregnancy riskier and steps can be taken to minimise those risks.

iv. Women with PCOS should ensure that they have a period at least once every 3 months. Some women with PCOS do not menstruate for long periods of time, sometimes many months, sometimes even years. The problem with this is that the endometrial lining can continue to grow without ever being shed. Hence abnormal changes can occur, which can lead to an increase in the risk of developing cancer of the endometrial lining. The easiest way to remedy this is to induce a withdrawal bleed by taking a progesterone (such as *Norethisterone* 5mg three times daily) for 10-14 days. Once stopped, the endometrial lining is destabilised and the endometrial lining is shed – the woman has a period. Always ensure that you are not pregnant before doing this.

v. When patients with PCOS are stimulated with *Clomid*, there is an increased risk of Ovarian Hyper-stimulation Syndrome (too many follicles stimulated in the ovaries). Stimulation with FSH in women with PCOS undergoing IVF/ICSI/IUI is like an all or nothing phenomenon. You can stimulate with a low dose of FSH and nothing happens. You increase the dose, then increase it again and still nothing happens – in other words no follicles are produced. You increase it a tiny bit more and "wham" – suddenly tens of follicles appear and the risk of OHSS becomes a reality. So great care is required when stimulating PCOS patients, particularly with FSH.

Finally – If you have PCOS - consider *Inofolic*

Inofolic is the brand name for a naturally occurring substance called myo-inositol combined with folic acid. It is taken orally, usually 2 sachets per day. Myo-inositol has found to be necessary for insulin modulation, particularly relevant for patients with PCOS who have insulin resistance. There is evidence that women with PCOS benefit from *Inofolic* in the following manner:

i. Improvement of fertility – improves menstrual cycle and improves ovulation rate.

ii. In women undergoing fertility treatment, it may be beneficial with regard to the pregnancy rates

iii. May reduce the testosterone level, and other abnormal blood tests to improve insulin resistance. Hence, studies show an improvement in acne and hirsutism (excess body hair).

iv. May help in reducing weight, blood pressure and harmful cholesterol.

Inofolic is available to buy over the internet on the Pharmasure website (www.inofolic.org.uk).

What are the author's views on *Inofolic*?

Since this is a naturally occurring substance with no side effects in any of the studies, why wouldn't you try it if you had PCOS? Additionally, since it contains folic acid – this has the additional benefit of reducing the risk of spina bifida in any subsequent pregnancy as well.

So the message is:

i.   Obese women with PCOS should be encouraged to lose weight – it will help with cycle control, improve fertility, reduce hirsutism (excess body hair) and help with acne.

ii.   You may have polycystic ovaries on ultrasound scan, but if you have regular cycles with ovulation with no androgenic features (excess facial or body hair/acne) you do NOT have polycystic ovarian SYNDROME.

iii. *Clomid* is a good first line treatment in women with PCOS to help them ovulate. This should be done with regular ultrasound scans (known as Follicle Tracking) to monitor ovarian follicles, give information on timing of ovulation (and therefore sexual intercourse) and ensure no cysts develop.

iv.   If you are already ovulating there is no point in using *Clomid* which might even be detrimental to your chances of conceiving.

v.   If you have PCOS, make sure you have a withdrawal bleed (period) at least once every 3 months unless you are on other hormones that stop your periods (like the contraceptive injection, or the Mirena coil).

vi.   If *Clomid* does not work after 6-9 months of trying, then ovulation induction with FSH is the next step.

vii. *Inofolic i*s a relatively new treatment option for women with PCOS that is free of side effects and is worth considering.

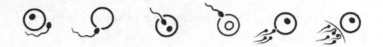

CHAPTER 9B

Endometriosis

Endometriosis is associated with reduced fertility and pelvic pain.

What is it?
First of all, patients often ask "what is endometriosis?" Despite being diagnosed with it and then told that they have the disease, they do not really understand what it is. In the broadest of layman's terms, endometriosis is essentially the lining of the womb (endometrium) existing and growing outside the womb. This means that in younger women in every cycle that goes by, the endometrium or lining of the womb grows thicker and then sheds as a period or menstrual loss. At the same time any other endometrium (endometriosis) outside the womb and dotted about the pelvis will also grow and shed, causing little bleeds – this can cause "scar" tissue and adhesions (sticky strands) which can then potentially damage the ovaries and fallopian tubes. Also, any scar tends to contract which can cause pulling between ovaries, tubes, and even the bowel – this can result in everything getting stuck together. So the tubes get blocked, the ovaries get covered and sometimes then cannot release eggs properly and patients become infertile AND get

pain – pelvic pain which is usually worse during a period and pain during sex.

What causes it?
There are many theories, but the truth is that nobody really knows.

How is it diagnosed?
If a young woman presents with awful pelvic pain, pain on sexual intercourse, then endometriosis should always be considered. From a gynaecologist's point of view, there are 4 pathological conditions that give a young woman pain in her pelvis:

i.   Pregnancy – ectopic pregnancy (pregnancy in the tube) or miscarriage
ii. Pelvic infection – which can cause tubal blockage, pus and abscesses within the pelvis
iii. Ovarian cysts – but these generally need to be 5cm or more in diameter
iv. ENDOMETRIOSIS

Other common non-gynaecological reasons for pelvic pain include constipation and cystitis (bladder infection). If the pregnancy test is negative, the swabs show no evidence of infection, and the ultrasound scan of the pelvis shows no cysts... then endometriosis must be considered.

The best way to diagnose endometriosis is to have a laparoscopy (keyhole surgery) – which is basically a fibre-optic camera usually placed through your tummy button (umbilicus) to look inside your pelvis. You need to be put to sleep for this (general anaesthesia). At the same time, the surgeon can surgically treat endometriosis by excising it, burning it off, or using a laser to remove it. Sometimes, endometriosis presents as "chocolate cysts" in one or both ovaries. It is possible to remove these cysts with keyhole surgery, although there is chance that by excising such cysts, healthy (egg producing) ovarian tissue can also be destroyed in the process.

An ultrasound scan of the pelvis can also help with the diagnosis, but can generally only be used to see "chocolate cysts" of the ovaries. It will not necessarily see the patches of endometriosis that are seen with a laparoscope – so a normal ultrasound scan does NOT exclude endometriosis.

How does endometriosis cause infertility and how common is it?

Endometriosis can block the fallopian tubes, stopping sperm getting up to the egg. It can cover the ovaries in adhesions, preventing the proper release of eggs into the tubes, as well destroying ovarian tissue. It causes a general "inflammatory" environment within the pelvis which is thought to reduce the chance of pregnancy. Finally, if the pelvis is distorted and sex is painful, the frequency of intercourse may decline, affecting fertility.

Whilst endometriosis can cause reduced fertility, it is also true that many women who have endometriosis successfully conceive naturally. So a diagnosis of endometriosis does not equate to an inability to have children. I have on many occasions seen endometriosis at laparoscopy in women having sterilisations because they do not want more children! That having been said, endometriosis does appear to be present in a significant number of women who have problems getting pregnant. Some authorities have inferred that endometriosis is present in as many as 20-65% of infertile women. However, remember that it is also true that many women with proven fertility also have endometriosis.

Can endometriosis be cured and how is it treated?

Once the diagnosis is made, endometriosis can certainly be effectively treated but it may well return if the woman is still having menstrual cycles. The growing and shedding of the endometrial tissue whether in the womb or outside the womb (as in endometriosis) is driven by oestrogen produced by the ovaries. Therefore when a woman becomes menopausal and the ovaries stop working, endometriosis gets better. If the ovaries are removed (often with the womb i.e. a hysterectomy), then endometriosis gets better. Oddly, when a woman becomes pregnant, because there is no menstruation (and no variation up and down of oestrogen levels), endometriosis gets better.

So to treat endometriosis, doctors often will give hormonal treatment that stops the ovaries producing oestrogen, which in turn stops the menstrual cycle (no growing and shedding of the lining of the womb), which in turn stops the growth of endometriosis. The trouble with giving hormone treatment is that if you stop the menstrual cycle you will also stop the woman getting pregnant. So, the combined oral contraceptive pill can be used often taken back to back for 3 months (so 3 packets in a row followed by a 7 day break when a withdrawal bleed occurs). I have previously introduced you to GNRHa (Gonadotrophin Release Hormone analogue) which is an injection usually given just under the skin that downregulates the production of your own fertility hormones. This therefore makes you temporarily menopausal and by stopping the production of oestrogen will help to treat endometriosis. This treatment is usually very good in sorting out the pain associated with endometriosis and will stop your periods. It is most often given in the form of a monthly injection (Prostap or Zoladex) for 4-6 months at a time. Side effects can include "hot flushes" as experienced when a woman gets to the menopause and thinning of bones if used for too long.

The alternative treatment is to have endometriosis surgically removed. This is usually done with keyhole surgery (laparoscopic excision). Mild endometriosis can be treated by a general gynaecologist, but if the endometriosis is severe it is better for any surgical treatment to be carried out by laparoscopic surgeon who specialises in the surgical treatment of endometriosis. This is because the surgery can be quite complex.

Does treating endometriosis help with fertility if you are trying to conceive naturally?

Firstly, remember that many women who have endometriosis still manage to get pregnant and have babies with no problems. If however, you have been trying to conceive for 1-2 years with no success, there is evidence that keyhole *surgical treatment of both mild and severe endometriosis helps* with spontaneous conception. However, there is *no* evidence to suggest that hormone treatment of endometriosis improves the conception rate in women trying to get pregnant naturally.

Does treating endometriosis help to improve success rates if you are having IVF?

If you are having IVF, there is some evidence that prescribing hormone treatment (GNRHa – *Zoladex* or *Prostap*) for 3 to 6 months before your IVF treatment can help improve pregnancy rates.

There is NO established benefit in surgically treating mild endometriosis before your IVF treatment cycle, although it *may* be considered.

If your ovaries are affected with endometriosis, for example you have an "Endometrioma" (Chocolate Cyst) there is NO good evidence to suggest removing it prior to IVF improves outcome even if it is greater than 3cm in size. This may be because removal of the Endometrioma may also destroy good ovarian tissue. However, many women will have removal of such lesions because they have other symptoms like pelvic pain.

If you have "deep endometriosis" (severe nodular lesions in the pelvis), there is NO GOOD EVIDENCE that surgical excision of these lesions before IVF will improve pregnancy rates.

If you want more information, then Google – "Management of women with endometriosis", ESHRE (European Society of Human Reproduction and Embryology) guideline.

Does IUI improve pregnancy rates in Mild Endometriosis compared to trying naturally?

The simple answer is "Yes". In women with mild endometriosis and infertility, as long as the fallopian tubes are open there is evidence that stimulated IUI increases the pregnancy rate.

So the message is:

1. Endometriosis is very common and there should be a low threshold for diagnostic laparoscopy to make the diagnosis.
2. Many women with endometriosis get pregnant and have children and never know that they have it.
3. Surgical treatment of endometriosis appears to help

women get pregnant naturally, but does not seem to help improve pregnancy rates if you are having IVF.

4. Hormonal treatment of endometriosis does not seem to help get women pregnant naturally, but hormonal treatment prior to IVF may help increase pregnancy rates.

5. Stimulated IUI cycles in women with endometriosis improve the pregnancy rates.

6. Pregnancy helps endometriosis.

7. If you have pelvic pain/pain on intercourse with no explanation, DO NOT be fobbed off. Request a laparoscopy to confirm the diagnosis of endometriosis.

8. If you have moderate or severe endometriosis – make sure that the gynaecologist who does your surgery specialises in endometriosis.

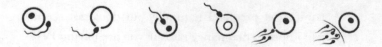

CHAPTER 10

Male Infertility / Donor Sperm

A third of the time, it is Male Infertility that is the cause of the inability of a woman to have a child.

What is a Normal Sperm Count?
The table below sets out what is a normal sample every time a man ejaculates (please see explanation for the table in Chapter 4). If the values are less than those shown there may be a potential problem. However, do not despair because there is now plenty that can be done.

World Health Organisation (2010) – normal values for Semen Samples:

Volume per ejaculate	1.5ml
Concentration	15 million sperm/ml
Progressive Motility	32%
Normal Forms	4%

At birth a woman has a set number of eggs and these reduce in number as time passes until the menopause, at which point they are completely depleted. On the other hand, men continue to produce a new batch of sperm every 3 to 4 months for many years and in fact fatherhood has on occasions been achieved by old-age pensioners.

Commonly used terms:

Azoospermia – no sperm seen on semen analysis

Oligospermia – reduced number of sperm seen on semen analysis

Teratospermia – abnormal looking sperm on semen analysis

What can impair the production of sperm?

In the event of a poor sperm sample, a repeat sample should be arranged. This is because a simple flu-like illness or sore throat can result in a temporary reduction in quality and concentration of sperm. After the illness, a repeat count preferably 3 months later may show a completely normal semen sample.

Avoid recreational drugs (for example – marijuana, heroin) since they can adversely affect sperm production. **Anabolic steroids may build big muscles but they trash the testicles.**

Alcohol can impair the production of sperm (even moderate drinking of 10 units per week) and cessation of drinking can make a difference, although it is important to allow time for improvement (at least 3 months).

Likewise, cigarette smoking reduces fertility for him and her, so it's important to stop. Obesity and related diabetes, or any chronic illness for that matter, can impair sperm production – so lose weight and seek comprehensive treatment for any ongoing illness.

Cycling – there have been reported cases of men spending too much time on the saddle who end up with impaired sperm samples and this reverses when they stop cycling. If the

testicles are exposed to too much heat for example, tight-fitting
trousers/tight underpants or too many hot baths, there may be
impairment of sperm production.

What medical reasons are there for an impaired sperm count?

Undescended Testes

Some men suffer from undescended testicles or "cryptorchid-
ism" to give it its proper medical title. About 3% of male
infants have no palpable testicles in the scrotal sac at birth,
although most of those have descended by the age of 1 year
old.

Some male children have "retractile" testes that can be
milked down into the scrotum where they remain for a few sec-
onds before springing back up. Whereas a truly undescended
testicle can sometimes be milked down, but will immediately
spring back. The former can be treated with an injection of
Hcg (Human chorionic gonadotrophin) which will in most
cases cause the retractile testes to descend – the undescended
testes will not respond and surgery (known as "orchidopexy")
is required. Men who have had 1 undescended testis tend to be
fertile, albeit with a reduced sperm count. Men with a history
of both testes undescended are at risk of infertility. It is also
important to note men with a history of undescended testes
are at greater risk of testicular cancer particularly if they do
not have surgery before the age of 10.

Viral Illness

Mumps can cause an "orchitis" (infection /inflammation of

the testicles) that can result in infertility. Hence the MMR vaccine protects against this.

STDs (sexually transmitted disease)

Not only can chlamydia cause blockage of the fallopian tubes in women, but infection can also cause blockage/damage to the male tubes (epididymis and vas) carrying sperm from the testicle to the penis as well as damage to the testicle itself. Other STDs such as gonorrhoea, which is thankfully less common now than it used to be, can also cause blockage and infertility. Hence the advice for young men and women – *any doubt, use a condom if in a new relationship or having casual sex.*

Varicose Veins of the Scrotum (Varicocele)

Varicose veins in the scrotal sac or varicoceles occur in up to 20% of the male population and feel like a bunch of worms in the scrotum – so they are common. What is interesting is that varicoceles are present in 30-40% of men attending fertility clinics and there is some evidence that they are associated with subfertility. That having been said, many men with varicoceles are fertile. The whole issue about treatment is controversial and there is no overwhelming evidence that surgery /treatment improves male fertility.

Trauma/Chemotherapy/Radiotherapy

Trauma is an obvious cause for permanent damage to the testicles and care should be taken when playing contact sports in particular.

If a patient has cancer and needs chemotherapy or radiotherapy, it is likely to affect their fertility and **they should at least be made aware of the possibility of giving sperm samples** *that can be frozen and then stored for future use before any such treatment.*

Obstruction or Absence of the Male Tubes

About 50% of men with azoospermia (no sperm in the semen sample) actually have normal sperm production in the testicles but there is a blockage preventing the sperm from exiting. This can be due to blockage of the sperm tubes (epididymis/vas) due to infection or previous vasectomy, or failure of the sperm tubes to ever develop (known as congenital absence of the vas deferens – CAVD). About 66% of men with absence of the vas deferens carry the cystic fibrosis gene and therefore may require testing for this to make sure that they cannot pass it on to their children.

Anti-sperm Antibodies (ASAs)

On occasions when a semen analysis is carried out and the sample is looked at under the microscope, clumping together of the sperm is seen under the microscope, indicating the presence of antibodies. These antibodies can be tested for. Antibodies to the sperm are likely to affect motility and perhaps fertilisation. At least 50% of men who have had a vasectomy will develop antibodies against their own sperm, but also infection, trauma, and the CAVD (Congenital Absence of the Vas Deferens) can cause antibodies against the sperm to form. It is NOT possible to wash off these antibodies and the best option for men with antibodies is to have IVF with ICSI. The concentration of anti-sperm antibodies does not affect success rates and birth rates using ICSI in men with ASAs are the same when compared to couples having ICSI when there are no male infertility problems. Clinicians used to use steroids to treat this – although these days most couples will opt for ICSI.

Idiopathic Male Factor Infertility (nobody knows)
About 50% of time no reason can be found for abnormal sperm and it is therefore labelled "idiopathic" – this is essentially akin to "Unexplained Infertility". Nobody knows why. Fortunately it can treated with IVF/ICSI.

If I have Male Factor Infertility… what can be done about it?

Simple everyday steps
Clearly the first simple steps are to avoid drugs, smoking, alcohol, obesity, tight-fitting underwear, excessive cycling. Ensure protection against STDs – use a condom. Get vaccinated with MMR early in your life. Wear loose-fitting clothes. Don't sit in hot baths for too long.

Anti-oxidants
In some of the harm to sperm is caused by "Oxidative Damage". This is damage to the DNA of the sperm by environmental pollution (e.g. traffic fumes, toxins in heavy industry, cigarette smoking) and environmental radiation. It therefore makes sense to include "anti-oxidants" in your diet to combat this and potentially improve the quality of your sperm. Hence, I often get asked if there is any evidence with regard to the taking of supplements like Zinc, Selenium, Vitamins B, C, E, and Co-enzyme Q10. The answer is that there is no absolute conclusive evidence. However, recently a new tablet was launched called *Condensyl*. This appears to boost the body's

natural anti-oxidant defence and subsequently may achieve a better pregnancy rate. Clinical studies thus far have indicated an improvement in pregnancy rates in couples who had previously been resistant to IVF and ICSI. It is thought that the use of *Condensyl* may also help in achieving natural conception in couples who have been struggling. Since men produce a new batch of sperm every 3-4 months, the advice is that you need to take the *Condensyl* daily for 4 months to achieve the best sperm result.

Varicose veins (Varicocele) of the scrotum
Again the evidence is not entirely clear and there are plenty of men with varicoceles who have fathered children. In the UK most surgical treatment is aimed at those who have symptoms, rather than to improve the sperm count especially when IVF/ICSI is available if the sperm count is low.

Chemotherapy/Radiotherapy
If at all possible, have sperm samples collected and frozen to be stored for future use ***prior*** to any treatment. This means the ability in the future to have children is preserved.

Overcoming obstruction of the male tubes (Vasectomy)

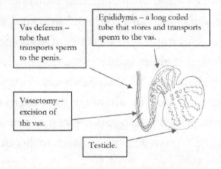

Vasectomy ("the snip") is essentially division of the vas or sperm tube. Sperm continues to be made by the testicle but cannot be transported beyond the surgically induced blockage.

If a man who has had a vasectomy meets a new partner and they wish to have their own children, there are a number of possible solutions:

1. Surgical Reversal of vasectomy (re-joining of the vas). The earlier after vasectomy that this reversal is done the better. More than 90% of men will have motile sperm in the ejaculate within 1 year of the vasectomy reversal but the ultimate goal is to achieve pregnancy. The quote for the best pregnancy rate is about 76% within 3 years of reversal. The longer the time gap between the vasectomy and its reversal the worse the pregnancy rate. The quoted figures are about a 50% pregnancy rate if the reversal is carried out within 10 years, 25% if the reversal is carried over 10 years from the original vasectomy.

   A problem with vasectomy is that 50-80% of men develop antibodies against their own sperm – Anti-Sperm Antibodies (ASAs) – these antibodies can cause clumping and affect the motility of the sperm as well as make it difficult for the sperm to interact with the egg – affecting fertilisation. Treatment options include the use of steroids which dampen down the immune system and so reduce the antibody number, OR consider IUI/IVF/ICSI.

2. Surgical Sperm Retrieval:
   PESA (Percutaneous Epidydimal Sperm Aspiration)
   TESE/TESA (Testicular Sperm Extraction/Aspiration)
   MESA (MicroEpididydimal Sperm Aspiration)

All 3 of these techniques involve either using a needle or a small incision to obtain sperm proximal to the vasectomy blockage. However, limited amounts of sperm are obtained and the procedure must be undertaken then with ICSI where only 1 good sperm is required and injected per egg collected from the female partner.

Surgical Sperm Retrieval

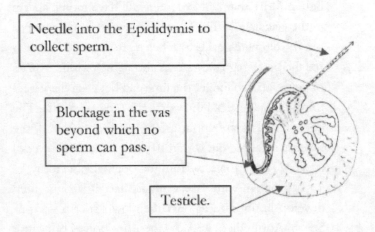

Needle into the Epididymis to collect sperm.

Blockage in the vas beyond which no sperm can pass.

Testicle.

Prior to the SSR, the patient needs to have shaved the scrotum. The procedure is usually done under local anaesthesia often with intravenous sedation and intravenous analgesia (painkillers). There is a risk of infection, bleeding, and bruising and it is sensible to wear supportive underwear following the procedure (no boxer shorts). Aspirin can increase the amount of bleeding and it is therefore sensible not to take aspirin either before or after the SSR.

SSR can be used to obtain sperm following a vasectomy, but also in cases where there is blockage for other reasons, or if there is an absent vas (as in CAVD – congenital absence of the vas deferens). In the latter case, it is sensible for the patient to have testing of his chromosomes particularly to ensure no evidence of cystic fibrosis carrier status (in other words, he carries the gene but does not have the disease).

Other screening blood tests will include HIV, Hepatitis B and C, and usually FSH. FSH or Follicle Stimulating Hormone stimulates the production of sperm in the testicles. If this is within the normal range, it is more likely that SSR will be more successful. On the other hand if it is abnormal, it is less likely that the testicles will be producing sperm and so SSR is less likely to be successful and donor sperm may be a more sensible option.

What happens if I cannot get an erection?
About 20% of the time, this is because of psychological problems like anxiety and depression. The rest of the time there is a physical cause. These includes diabetes, multiple sclerosis, spinal cord injury, or previous surgery to the groin area (for example prostate surgery). Some drugs, for example blood pressure tablets, can also be responsible. It is sensible to see your GP regarding this as a first line. Treatment is usually with a well-known medication like "*Viagra*". If this does not work referral to hospital is appropriate.

What is Retrograde Ejaculation?
Retrograde ejaculation occurs during sex, when instead of the sperm coming out of the end of the penis, it goes into the bladder (the reservoir for urine). This results in only a small amount of sperm being produced externally. The best way to determine the diagnosis is to collect a urine sample after ejaculation. If

sperm are seen in the urine, the diagnosis is made. This does make it difficult to achieve a pregnancy naturally, however, if required the sperm can be collected from the urine and used for IVF/ICSI to achieve pregnancy.

If all else fails, what else can I do? DONOR SPERM

Donor sperm is available from various clinics up and down the UK as well as 2 other sources of donor sperm:

i.   European Sperm Bank which is based in Denmark (www.esb.com)

ii.   Xytex which is based in the USA (www.xytex.com)

Sperm from these overseas sources have a vast selection of donor sperm available to meet the personal criteria required in terms of characteristics of the donors. In addition and reassuringly they also comply with UK laws regarding screening and quarantining.

Donor sperm can be used not only in the absence of sperm of a partner, but also in cases when the male partner has an inherited condition that the couple do not want to pass on to their children.

Donor sperm can also be used by same-sex couples, or indeed a single woman who wishes to have a baby but has no male partner.

Donated sperm can used in either IUI or IVF cycles.

When donated sperm is used, your clinic must sort out various consents to enable legality of parenthood for:

i.   Married couples

ii.   Civil partners

iii. Women who are not married or in a civil partnership but have a male partner

iv. Women who are not married or in a civil partnership but have a female partner

Certainly, the sperm donor is NOT to be treated as the father of any child resulting from the use of his sperm in the treatment of others.

Can children conceived through the use of donor sperm access information about the donor?

The answer to this is yes, once the child is 18 years old (if the donation was made after April 2005). This information can be identifying information including name, date of birth, address, and physical appearance.

In addition, once 18 years old, an individual can also find out about donor-conceived genetic brothers or sisters – if both sides consent.

Can donors access information about their genetic offspring?

The answer is yes, but the information is anonymous – so they are made aware of the number, sex, date of birth, of people born as a result of their donation.

The Human Fertilisation & Embryology Authority (HFEA) keep a confidential register of all sperm, egg, and embryo donations. This includes information on ethnicity, physical appearance, occupation and interests. The register also includes information on all treatments and children born as a result of such treatments.

Should fertility units offer counselling regarding the use of donor sperm/eggs?

The answer is of course yes. Clinics should offer couples

counselling regarding all aspects of fertility, but particularly the use of donor sperm and eggs.

Further reading, particularly regarding the legal aspects of using donor sperm, can be found on the HFEA website at http://www.hfea.gov.uk.

So the message is:
1. Poor or absent sperm is responsible for one third of all cases of infertility.
2. The most important investigation for the male partner is the semen analysis or sperm count test.
3. Simple lifestyle changes like reduction of alcohol, stopping smoking, stopping drugs, prevention of STDs, and promotion of loose-fitting clothes can make a difference and are worth trying.
4. Consider *Condensyl* as an anti-oxidant to improve sperm quality.
5. If you have had a vasectomy or there is a blockage in the sperm tubes, sperm can still be retrieved using a surgical sperm retrieval for use with ICSI.
6. If all else fails, you can still use donor sperm.
7. If you are in a same-sex female relationship, you can use donor sperm.
8. If you are a single woman, you can use donor sperm.

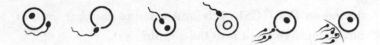

CHAPTER 11

Basic Embryology – What You Need To Know

A book on infertility and IVF would not be complete without some mention of the science behind Assisted Reproduction and how it relates to you in your attempts to have a child.

What is an embryologist and what do they do?

An embryologist is a highly trained and specialised scientist who works in the laboratory of IVF Units. They are essentially involved in everything from the basic sperm tests (semen analysis) to identification of eggs at egg collection, to the IVF/ICSI procedure itself when they are responsible for the fertilisation of the eggs, the culturing of the embryos, and the embryo transfer. They are responsible for the storage of sperm/eggs/embryos. Not only do they provide scientific expertise based in the laboratory but they also liaise and provide information to infertile couples both before, during, and after a fertility treatment.

What happens during the development of an embryo

during an IVF/ICSI cycle and when is the best time to put an embryo back into the womb?

Day 0 – Egg collection is carried out and the eggs prepared for IVF or ICSI. Sperm is prepared either from a thawed frozen sample or a fresh sample. In IVF up to 150,000 sperm are placed with each egg retrieved. In ICSI 1 sperm is injected into each egg retrieved.

Day 1 – The embryologist carries out a fertilisation check to ensure the formation of embryos. The couple are usually contacted to inform them of the number of fertilised eggs (embryos).

Day 2 – The embryos have started to divide and are now composed of between 2-4 cells. At this stage the embryo can either be transferred into the womb (Embryo Transfer – ET) or frozen for a Frozen Embryo Transfer (FET) at a later date or be allowed to continue to develop.

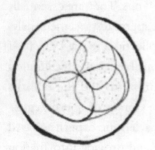

> **Day 2 Embryo**
> – 4 cell stage.
> Can replace into
> the womb.

Day 3 – The embryo continues to divide and is now composed of 6-8 cells. At this stage the embryo can either be transferred into the womb (ET) or frozen for a future FET or be allowed to continue to develop to day 5 (Blastocyst stage).

Day 4 – At this stage the embryo is called a Morula. It is just a cluster of cells and as such it is blurry and difficult to grade.

Day 5 – The embryo reaches the "Blastocyst" stage. Now the embryo has an "inner cell mass" which will develop into the baby, and the "trophectoderm" which develops into the placenta or afterbirth. The embryo expands to have a fluid-filled cavity and the embryo is encased within a shell through which it must hatch in order to implant into the lining of the womb.

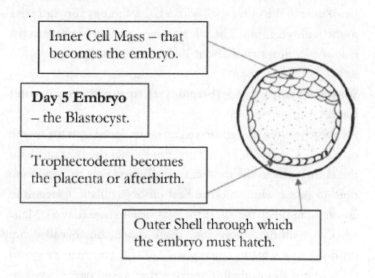

Inner Cell Mass – that becomes the embryo.

Day 5 Embryo
– the Blastocyst.

Trophectoderm becomes the placenta or afterbirth.

Outer Shell through which the embryo must hatch.

The embryologist grades each embryo to determine the best one or two to place into the womb. As can be seen from the above diagram, there is an outer shell around the embryo from which the embryo needs to hatch in order to implant into the lining of the womb. If the outer shell looks tough, or there is a history of previously failed implantation (especially in the over 40s), then the embryologist can facilitate "hatching" by making a small hole in the outer shell with a laser:

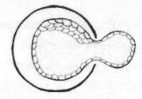

Day 5 Embryo – hatching through its outer shell.

Are there any risks with Assisted Hatching?
If the embryologist undertakes assisted hatching by making a small hole in the outer shell with a laser, there is very little risk to the embryo, if any. There is however, a slight increase in the risk of identical twins (about 1%).

Why wait until day 5 (blastocyst) to put the embryo(s) back?
As already stated, the embryos can be replaced into the womb on day 2/3 or day 5. There is no doubt that the best place for the embryos is in the mother's womb, however the optimum time to judge which are the best embryos likely to result in an ongoing pregnancy is at the blastocyst stage (day 5). Many embryos will die before they reach day 5, but because you do not know which embryos will survive you may carry out embryo transfer using the embryos that would never have survived until day 5. Since only the strongest and best embryos make it to blastocyst and it is these that are replaced into the womb, it is not surprising that pregnancy rates have gone up with blastocyst replacement.

Following on from this, if your egg collection and subsequent fertilisation only results in 2 embryos, it is sensible to have embryo transfer on day 2/3 since there is no choice between embryos and no advantage in waiting until day 5 to replace them. However, if you have more embryos to choose from, wait until day 5 to determine the fittest and the highest grade embryo(s) to replace.

What is an embryoscope and how does it help in choosing the best embryos?

The "embryoscope" is a cutting-edge embryo incubator that essentially employs time lapse photography to film the progress of the developing embryos. A photograph is taken every 15 minutes so that development of each embryo from the time of fertilisation to the time of embryo transfer is recorded. Hence, when each embryo is ready to be placed back into the womb not only can the embryo be graded according to what it looks like now, but also the development of each embryo from the earliest stages can be assessed. If there has been abnormal development noted by reviewing images from the embryoscope, then that embryo is less likely to produce a viable pregnancy. On the other hand if the embryo has shown normal development as witnessed by the embryoscope, then it is more likely to yield a viable pregnancy. In this way the embryoscope provides more information on how to choose the best embryos for embryo transfer to improve the chance of a positive pregnancy test and ongoing pregnancy.

What is Embryo Glue?

The embryos can be placed into "Embryo Glue" prior to their transfer into the womb. This is a great marketing name, but is certainly nothing like glue. It is thought the "glue" facilitates communication between cells and is helpful for the process of implantation. Some embryologists feel that there is a small advantage to using this prior to embryo transfer.

Embryologists and Sperm Assessment and Preparation

Embryologists carry out semen analysis to determine whether the sperm sample is adequate for IUI or IVF or ICSI, and of course they prepare the sperm for each of these treatments and in the case of ICSI inject the sperm directly into the collected egg. Sperm preparation involves washing the sperm to remove any dead sperm or debris, then centrifuging or spinning the sperm cells down to increase the concentration. In patients having ICSI, they can also carry out a procedure called IMSI.

What is IMSI?

IMSI stands for Intracytoplasmic Morphological Sperm Injection. In English, this means that when the embryologist is looking for the best single sperm to use for injection, they use a special microscope that is x6000 more powerful to assess each sperm. In this way tiny defects in the sperm that would not ordinarily have been seen are detected and only "perfect" sperm used to inject into the egg. Hence IMSI is a useful selection tool for the embryologist in choosing the best sperm.

What is "DNA Fragmentation" of the sperm?

The head of the sperm contains genetic material called DNA which needs to remain intact. If this genetic material or DNA gets damaged or "fragmented", it may cause problems with subsequent embryos that are produced, both in terms of implantation and possible miscarriage. A "DNA fragmentation test" is essentially a method of looking at the sperm head to determine if there is any genetic damage or fragmentation.

When is IMSI useful?

IMSI is recommended in couples in whom there is recurrent implantation failure, failed ICSI, or indeed in sperm samples with many of the sperm showing an abnormal form or shape. In addition, IMSI can be used to choose the best sperm in patients with elevated sperm DNA fragmentation.

So the message is:

1. The embryologist is a highly trained scientist working in IVF units who is responsible for all the laboratory aspects of IVF and ICSI.

2. If you have enough embryos, embryo transfer at the Blastocyst stage, day 5, yields higher pregnancy rates.

3. Consider assisted hatching if your embryologist recommends it, particularly if you are over 40 years old or had previous implantation failures.

4. The embryoscope is useful for better selection of embryos to be transferred.

5. Consider IMSI if there has been previous implantation failure in an ICSI cycle when the sperm analysis has shown many sperm with abnormal shape or form. Also consider IMSI when there is elevated sperm DNA fragmentation.

GOOD LUCK IN YOUR JOURNEY!

About the author:

Dr Watermeyer is a Fellow of the Royal College of Obstetricians and Gynaecologists, as well as a Member of the Royal College of General Practitioners. He has been a consultant in Obstetrics and Gynaecology at the Royal Glamorgan Hospital since 2007. Sean qualified as a doctor in 1990 and initially served in the RAF in the UK, Germany and Bosnia completing his general practice training during that time.

After leaving the Forces, and working as a GP, Sean decided to retrain in Obstetrics and Gynaecology, following the birth of his first son when he was unimpressed by the actions of an Obstetric Registrar who was looking after his wife and unborn child in labour.

In addition to his NHS duties, he carries out some private work at the Vale Hospital, Hensol and The Centre for Reproduction and Gynaecology (CRGW), Llantrisant, Nr.Cardiff – a highly regarded Fertility Unit.

Sean met his beloved wife, Alison in Germany where she was also a serving officer. They have been married for over twenty years and have three children.

Personal Notes

Personal Notes